Dat

615.82 BRE
Brennan, Richard.
Mind and body stress relief
with the Alexander techniq...

PALM BEACH COUNTY
LIBRARY SYSTEM
3650 SUMMIT BLVD.
WEST PALM BEACH, FL 33406

Mind and Body Stress Relief with the Alexander Technique

Richard Brennan

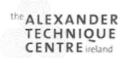

The Alexander Technique Centre, Ireland

Kirkullen Lodge, Tooreeny, Moycullen, Co Galway, Ireland

Phone: +353 91 555800

Web: www.alexander.ie

Email: info@alexander.ie

About the author

Richard Brennan found relief from painful back problems and sciatica after discovering the Alexander Technique in 1984. He found the Technique so effective that he decided to undertake a three year full time teacher training approved by the Society of Teachers of the Alexander Technique UK, qualifying in 1989.

Richard aims to make the Alexander Technique accessible to a wide audience. He has written six books on the Alexander Technique, which are translated into eight languages and are on sale world-wide. He has been featured in many newspapers and magazines including The Irish Times, The Sunday Tribune, The Irish Examiner, Cosmopolitan, Hello Magazine and Home and Country. He has appeared on BBC I & RTE 1 and been featured on BBC Radios 4 & 5, as well as on numerous local radio stations around Ireland and the UK. He travels extensively around Europe and USA, giving talks and courses on the Technique.

Richard is Director of the only Alexander Technique Teacher Training College in Ireland, which he founded in 1998. The training college is approved by the Society of Teachers of Alexander Technique (STAT) and the Irish Society of Alexander Technique Teachers (ISATT). He is co-founder and past president of ISSAT.

Other titles by Richard Brennan

- *The Alexander Technique - Natural Poise for Health* (1991, 1993, 1995, 1997) ISBN 1-86204-046-X
- *The Alexander Technique Manual* (1996, 2004) ISBN 1-85906-163-X

- *Mind & Body Stress Relief with the Alexander Technique* (1998) ISBN 0-7225-3504-X

- *Stress - The Alternative Solution* (2000) ISBN 0-572-02609-9

- *The Alexander Technique Workbook* (1992, 2011) ISBN 978-1-84340-594-8

- *Change Your Posture, Change Your Life: How the Power of the Alexander Technique Can Combat Back Pain, Tension and Stress* (Due for publication in January 2012) ISBN 978-1780280240

While the author of this work has made every effort to ensure that the information contained in this book is as accurate and up to date as possible, the application of it to particular circumstances depends on many factors. Therefore it is recommended that readers always consult a qualified medical specialist for individual advice.

The Alexander Technique should not be used as an alternative to orthodox medicine, but rather to complement it. If in doubt, see your doctor.

The publishers regret that they have not been able to trace or acknowledge the copyright holders of the works by Nadine Stair and Sibyl Partridge. They will be happy to acknowledge the holders in future editions if they are notified.

Alexander Technique Centre, Ireland

www.alexander.ie

© Richard Brennan 1998, 2011

Richard Brennan asserts the moral right to be identified as the author of this work

First published in print by Thorsons 1998
\An Imprint of HarperCollinsPublishers. A catalogue record for this book is available from the British Library
ISBN 978-1-94361-228-4

2011 electronic book version contains updated contact details, Chapter 9 (2008 trials), useful addresses and further reading sections.

All rights reserved. No part of this publication may be reproduced, stored in a retrieval system, or transmitted, in any form or by any means, electronic, mechanical, photocopying, recording or otherwise, without the prior permission of the publishers.

For Cara, Tim, Ciaran and Laoise

A human being is part of the whole called by us 'the Universe', a part limited in time and space. He experiences himself, his thoughts and feelings, as something separate from the rest; a kind of optical delusion of his consciousness. This delusion is a kind of prison for us, restricted to our personal desires and to affections for a few persons nearest to us. Our task must be to free ourselves from this prison by widening our circle of understanding and compassion to embrace all living creatures and the whole of nature and beauty.

Albert Einstein

Contents

Acknowledgements – xii

Introduction – 1

1 Stress and Quality of Life – 7

2 Principles of the Alexander Technique – 34

3 The Physical Effects of Stress – 57

4 Worry – 75

5 Anxiety – 95

6 Depression – 117

7 Stress and Emotions – 131

8 The Breath of Life – 142

9 The Freedom to Change – 155

Useful Addresses – 173

Further Reading – 178

Index – 181

Acknowledgements

First, I wish to express my sincere thanks to my wife Caroline, who corrected my first draft and gave me many ideas on how to improve the book. Secondly, to Sarah Widdecome for a thorough examination of the text and for putting the right punctuation in the right places. And thirdly to my editor Wanda Whiteley and her associates at Thorsons - Barbara Vesey, Jo Ridgeway, Paul Redhead - for helping to make the project as stress-free as possible from beginning to end. I should also like to thank Ed Brennan for his research help.

Introduction

This book sets out to explain how the Alexander Technique can alleviate physical stress and help to reduce mental and emotional stress as well. It may be particularly helpful to those suffering from depression, panic attacks, anxiety and worry, as it points the way to the simple but powerful technique that has already helped many thousands of people.

Woody Allen is quoted as having said, 'More than at any time in history, mankind faces a crossroads. One path leads to despair and utter hopelessness, the other to total extinction. Let's pray we have the wisdom to choose correctly!' This book is about another path, another choice, another way of being; one that offers hope and contentment to our children rather than the possible disasters that now face mankind in the form of stress-related illnesses and the global stresses that environmentalists have been warning about for decades.

F Matthias Alexander, the progenitor of the Technique, developed his unique method not only as a way of improving posture and physical health, but also as a route to freeing people from the 'fixed prejudices' and 'erroneous concepts' which prevent them from being truly happy. Like the great philosophers Socrates, Plato and Hippocrates, Alexander realized that there is an inseparable unity between the body, mind and emotions; he was convinced that mental stress will invariably lead to muscle tension and emotional instability, and vice versa.

Many view the Alexander Technique simply as a way of improving posture or of alleviating back pain. While it can be effective in both these respects, its full potential has still to be discovered by the majority of people.

I was asked to write this book on how the Alexander Technique can help those afflicted with stress just two weeks before commencing a four-month, round-the-world trip. My first reaction, therefore, was that this project could not have come at a more inconvenient time. The last things I needed were deadlines and the problem of trying to communicate with my London publishers from tropical islands halfway around the world. These two factors alone were bound to cause tension, and writing a book on how to reduce stress while being under stress myself did not make any sense, no matter which way I looked at it.

As the days passed, however, I began to realize that this could be a unique opportunity to study the effects that different types of stress have on people from very diverse cultures and lifestyles around the globe. It was also an excellent chance to examine whether or not Alexander's theories and philosophies, which were formed over 75 years ago, were still relevant. All I needed was to overcome my prevailing anxiety.

Once I was able to think calmly about my dilemma, the solution seemed very straightforward: I needed to negotiate more time to complete the book, and arrange to take a portable computer with me on my travels. Both of these requirements were met within a few hours.

My travels took me throughout Europe, to the US, Tahiti, Raratonga, Fiji, New Zealand, Australia and Hong Kong. Each country I visited was at a different stage of development and evolving at a different rate; as a consequence, parts of this book were written in modern hotels in California, where it was possible to order room service via the television's remote control, hardly moving a muscle, while other parts were composed on board a luxury ship cruising exotic South Pacific Islands, and still other parts were put together shortly after visiting simple Tahitian villages or taking part in the ancient kava ceremony in Fiji. In some of the places I visited, new technology was becoming available by the day, whereas in others life had changed little in the last thousand years - and the native people certainly had little or no concept of deadlines or book projects.

Because of the contrasting places I visited, my journey became a very surreal experience. One day I would be encountering people still living in houses made of banana leaves and sleeping on mud floors, with just enough food to feed themselves and their families for that day, and the next I would be in a modern city where people worked frantically in front of computer screens in high-rise office buildings or talking as fast as possible into their cellular telephones while stuck in heavily congested traffic. Because of these extreme contrasts, it became obvious to me that the people in these cities were under far more stress than their 'less civilized' counterparts, and as a result had less time to interact with each other. Although many of these people had both wealth and technology to help them in their daily lives, their manner seemed more abrupt and even hostile at times, and they seemed to be generally more miserable and self-centred. It was actually unusual to see them smiling - unless they were under the influence of alcohol! By contrast, in the 'less advanced' cultures the people were not nearly so goal-orientated; they laughed and smiled more often, and when they did so they beamed from ear to ear. These people were much more friendly, had time to sit and talk, were more easy-going and on the whole seemed happier and more fulfilled.

It appears to me that with all our modern advances we may indeed be less hungry and generally more comfortable, but on the whole we are more stressed and far less contented than the people living their lives in less technologically and economically sophisticated societies. To find answers in our search for a less stressful life, however, does not involve returning to a more 'primitive' existence, but taking the next step forward on our evolutionary path. The aim of the Alexander Technique, is to give us the choice of achieving a happier and less pressurized way of life without necessarily having to reduce our standard of living.

Even from the vantage point of the 1920s, Alexander could foresee that the world was heading towards the very serious problems apparent today. Even then it was clear that the increasing pace of life was having a harmful effect on mankind; today people are under a great deal more pressure, both at work and in their relationships at home, than ever before. There no longer seems to be enough time to enjoy the simple things in life, and as a result ill-health, unhappiness and worry often blight our quality of life.

The technique Alexander developed is a powerful method of releasing the mental and emotional tension that can often build up when we are under stress. Many of the numerous physical problems from which we suffer are caused directly by our harmful thought patterns, which can manifest as acute anxiety, worry, depression, boredom or irritability. Alexander devised his unique method as a way of combating the detrimental effects of stressful lifestyles which affect our psychological and emotional well-being. This book will help those trying to find a way of alleviating everyday stresses and strains, facing deadline after deadline at work or an erratic or traumatic emotional life at home, or feeling that their full potential as conscious and joyful human beings has yet to be achieved.

1
Stress and Quality of Life

We must learn to awaken and keep ourselves awake,
not by mechanical aids, but by an infinite expecta-
tion of the dawn, which does not forsake us in our
soundest sleep. I know of no more encouraging fact
than the unquestionable ability of man to elevate his
life by a conscious endeavour. It is something to be
able to paint a particular picture, or to carve a statue,
and so to make a few objects beautiful, but it is far
more glorious to carve and paint the very atmosphere
and medium through which we look, which morally
we can do. To affect the quality of the day, that is the
highest art.

Henry David Thoreau

Stress: A Way of Life?

'Improving the quality of life' appears to be one objective that everyone on this planet shares. It is the reason for all the technology and 'progress' over the centuries, and concerns us now more than ever before.

It is natural to want to find a happier and more contented way of living, and each of us chooses different ways in our search. Despite our efforts, however, it is often the case that the enjoyable times we experience become less frequent and shorter in duration the more we 'progress'. Surveys confirm this and report that a quarter of men and a third of the women suffer from anxiety or depression. It appears that the harder we strive for happiness the more it eludes us, and as a result we can feel angry and more disillusioned with life as time goes on. Despite all our obvious material gains, many of us suffer from a new affliction - chronic stress.

Stress is a problem that affects us physically, mentally, emotionally and spiritually. It can cause anxiety, which in extreme cases may permeate our whole existence until life is hardly worth living. It affects us physically in such a way that our whole system is constantly on 'red alert', ageing us before our time. It can even cause stress-related illnesses such as strokes and heart problems which can threaten life itself. Stress affects us mentally by over-stimulating the mind, eventually causing mental blocks or, conversely, an overactive mind which gives us little or no control over persistent unwanted thoughts, causing endless worry for no reason. It affects us emotionally because we can lose control of our anger and react irrationally, perhaps eventually damaging our relationships with family or friends. And it affects us spiritually by preventing us from being in contact with the peace and tranquillity that should be the very essence and foundation of our lives.

How often do we really pause for even a moment to see whether the path we have taken in life is actually making us more satisfied, fulfilled and contented - and if not, why not?

The Price We Pay for Progress

On the whole, society rarely measures progress in terms of how people feel, concentrating instead on our ability to accomplish certain tasks. In fact, we are now 25 times more productive than we were 150 years ago, and during this time the manner in which we live has changed more than at any other time in human history. With the introduction of time-saving technology we have been promised an easier lifestyle with more comfort and leisure time than ever before - yet is this really the case? From the way many of us rush around trying to keep appointments, meet important deadlines or reach impossible targets, it seems as if the very opposite is happening.

Even though it is obvious that we now live longer and are far more efficient than we used to be, when you add joy and fulfilment to the equation it is not at all clear that we have really achieved a better quality of life.

When we talk about progress we must consider all aspects of life, including - though this should be obvious - how much peace and happiness we feel. Despite the huge volume of technology now at our disposal, it seems that more people are suffering from continuous stress than perhaps at any other time. An increasing number of people are visiting their doctors when they find themselves trapped in an accelerated spiral of speed and stress which can manifest itself in chronic muscle tension, acute anxiety, fidgety or restless behaviour, or a distinct lack of peace of mind. Sleeping tablets or anti-depressants may present a short-term solution, but we need to find a more permanent answer that does not rely on the use of potentially addictive drugs, many of which lose their effect over a period of time.

If we feel stressed during our working day, adrenalin - which causes the brain to be in a state of excitation - remains in our system for many hours or even days afterwards, and as a result we are likely to have less patience than usual. When we arrive home, we may be more prone to anger or irritation than we otherwise would be. The increase in stress over recent years certainly takes a toll on marriage. The alarming divorce statistics - which don't take into account the escalating number of unmarried couples who separate, nor the increase in unwanted teenage pregnancies where the couple may not live together in the first place - reflect just one possible side-effect of rising stress levels.

> Current statistics that show over 50 per cent of marriages in the US and 40 per cent in the UK end in divorce.
>
> *Office for National Statistics, UK, 1995; US National Center for Health Statistics, 1994*

City Life and Work

Today, over half the population of the world lives in cities and has to cope with the incessant noise, pollution, overcrowded living conditions and traffic congestion that accompany city life. Even those people who are financially well off are not immune to the effects of stress in the city and therefore are not necessarily any happier than their less well off counterparts. In fact, it sometimes seems that the more material possessions a person has the more unhappy he or she becomes: perhaps this is because such people feel they have more to lose should they risk scaling down their work and financial commitments.

Modern society, in which money has become more important than health or education, is becoming more and more dehumanized;

an enormous number of homeless people wander the streets, while at the same time there is an increase in the number of people who own a second holiday home; tons of food are wasted each day, yet at the same time millions of children are starving to death. Many people today are angry, confused, depressed or frustrated, as their search for happiness is hampered by unseen obstacles. Although it is profoundly clear that materialism is not the answer, we continue to think that money will be the solution to our problems.

We are living in a strange world indeed, as an increasing number of us stare at a computer or television screen for a large proportion of our lives. This type of static posture tends to cause both physical and emotional stress.

Stress is also extremely infectious. Just as we are favourably affected when we come into contact with happy or lively people, and a smile or kind word can brighten up our day, so we will absorb stressful atmospheres and pick up other people's tension without realizing it. This causes us to become irritated with our family, friends or colleagues at work without knowing why. In fact, stress at work is now reaching crisis point, as people are given huge workloads to complete in impossibly brief time spans. There is a common underlying feeling that if we are not rushing around feeling panicked or overwhelmed then we are not being responsible. Many people I talk to have been subjected to unspoken pressures to get them to work extra hours. If they refuse, bosses and colleagues alike will imply that they are 'letting the side down' or 'not pulling their weight'. They are also aware that if they do not 'toe the line' their chances of promotion will be severely affected, or they may even lose their job. These fears are often caused by subtle, unspoken emotional pressures which can be very hard to ignore. There is also the pressure not to take time off even when genuinely ill. The stress we're likely to feel if we do take time off - or continue soldiering on - is thus likely to increase, leading to more chronic illness later on.

Hint

When coping with impossible deadlines we need to remember that no one has ever been reported as saying on their deathbed, 'I wish I'd spent more time at the office' or 'I wish I'd reached those business targets.'

The Costs of Stress

The penalties of stress on our society are enormous. Just stop for a moment to consider the following facts, taken from a book entitled Understanding Stress (Brockhampton Reference Series):

- In the US, the incidence of heart disease is increasing by 100 pecent every 10 years.
- In the US, 16,000 tons of aspirin and over 5 billion tranquillizers are consumed each year.
- In the US, the annual estimated medical cost of stress is over $1 billion.
- In the UK, 250,000 people die every year from heart attacks.
- In the UK, over 40 million working days are lost every year through illness directly related to stress. The cost to British industry is estimated at £1.5 billion each year.

These figures could easily double over the next 20 years. As we work harder and harder to improve our quality of life, the opposite is being achieved.

Recognizing Stress

It is important to distinguish between the constructive energy we feel when we face new challenges in life and the detrimental effects of continual stress over a long period of time. People talk of 'stress management', but as far as we can we need to *eliminate* as much stress from our lives as possible, rather than just learn how cope with it.

Although stress has very definite physical effects, such as high blood pressure or the production of specific hormones, we are usually unaware of these bodily changes. The way in which we detect stress in ourselves or others varies, but stress will often manifest in one of three visible ways: *worry, anxiety or depression.* These problems are so prevalent in our society that this book devotes a chapter to each.

The Vicious Circle of Stress

There are differing opinions throughout the medical profession as to the physical effects of stress. Some doctors believe that stress can cause high blood pressure and an increase in the level of fatty acids in the blood, which is a contributory cause of heart disease and hypertension. Others believe that excessive tension over a period of time causes a reduction in the body's own immune system defences, and as a result leaves us open to a wide range of diseases. Whichever way you look at it, stress is bad for your health.

Let's take the example of the habitual reaction which arises when we are running late for an appointment. Many of us respond by tensing our whole body, hunching our shoulders, clenching our teeth or arching our back. As we fear the consequences of being late, we are no longer in conscious control of our actions and may well act irrationally. If we are driving, we may even take unnecessary risks which could threaten our own or other people's lives. This in turn can make us even more stressed, and a vicious circle ensues. Our habitual reaction becomes so ingrained that we experience muscle tension even when we think we are relaxed. If this behaviour is allowed to persist over a period of time, we may end up suffering from one of the stress-related illnesses listed below:

- Asthma and other breathing problems
- Backache
- Neck problems
- Cardiac arrest (heart attack)
- Diabetes
- Digestive disorders
- Headaches and migraines
- Hypertension (high blood pressure)
- Skin complaints
- Fibromyalgia
- Ulcers
- ME and chronic fatigue
- Depression
- Panic attacks
- Increasingly goal-orientated attitudes (see Chapter 1, 'End Gaining')

Habitual Stress

The spiritual teacher Krishnamurti once said: "'It seems to me that the greatest stumbling block in life is this constant struggle to reach, to achieve, to acquire."' Certainly a great number of people who come to me for Alexander lessons seem to be suffering from stress, the root cause of which is an obsession with acquiring more and more material goods. Yet few people make the connection between the tendency to acquire and achieve and the uncomfortable symptoms of stress that they experience.

We treat life as though it were some kind of emergency, forgetting that in reality it is a very precious - and impermanent - gift. Although experiencing minimal amounts of stress now and again is quite normal, and indeed is a part of living, continual stress at work or at home can be detrimental to every area of life and is neither efficient nor useful in any way.

Being under stress in this way can become an ingrained habit, to the point where people become restless, nervous or worried when there is nothing to do. When we suffer from habitual stress, just waiting for the lift or being in a queue at the supermarket may be all it takes to annoy us. This has even come to be seen as normal human behaviour. As with so many other habits, we need determination if we are to break free of it.

The Causes of Stress

In order to start combating stress it is essential that we first understand what causes it and what it is doing to our body and mind.

Stress can be a response to external events and its causes are numerous and varied, but its effects will be moderated by our nature and constitution. When discussing stress, it is therefore helpful to consider both external and internal factors.

External Factors

The external factors are the many outside stimuli that our senses perceive. We are not always aware that certain external events are causing stress - for example we may feel agitated when road workers are using very loud machinery, but it is not until the noise stops and we feel relief that we realize that we were disturbed by it.

External factors include:

- Major life events: the death of a spouse, close friend or relative; divorce; imprisonment; personal injury or accident; a new job, losing a job; pregnancy or the birth of a baby; attending a new school; moving house and other circumstances that bring about significant changes in our lives

- Physical environment: anything unpleasant that we experience through our five senses - bright or flashing lights; loud or strange noises; heat or cold; unpleasant tastes or smells; confined places, etc.

- Daily problems: traffic; losing important documents or keys; car or household appliances not working; parking or speeding tickets and so on all fall into this category. Often, the more stressed we are the more likely that we will be to forget or lose things, and the more vigorously we will react when we do.

- Social interaction: impolite or rude behaviour, for example while driving, can be a source of stress. The more stressed our society becomes as a whole, the more likely we are to encounter aggressive behaviour from others. If we react to the stress of others the situation may escalate out of all proportion, as attested by the increase in cases of 'road rage'.

- Social restrictions: having to be on time for an appointment or to meet unreasonable deadlines; petty rules and regulations or 'red tape'. Again, the more wound-up we are the more we will react against the trivial restrictions placed on us and vice versa.

> Intrusive advertisements and flashing lights in cities and on television demand our attention and over-stimulate our neuro-muscular system.
>
> To add to this stress burden, the media continually report increasing violence and social disorder throughout the world; while it may be true that it is no longer safe to walk the streets in many modern cities, even in daylight, the reportage itself over-excites our fear responses, even when we are not actually in danger.

Internal Factors

Internal factors are determined by our own physiological make-up. They include the way we think and behave, and the reaction we have to certain situations, as well as our perception of life.

- Personality traits: long-term in-built tendencies which define a person's character, such as being a perfectionist, workaholic or habitually disorganized
- Negative thinking: the tendency to think the worst of oneself, others or events. People will be more prone to stress if they tend towards pessimism, self-criticism or being over-analytical.
- Lifestyle: lack of sleep or physical exercise, inadequate diet, too much caffeine and trying to fit too much into the day

- Mental perceptions: rigid ways of thinking, taking comments too personally or having unrealistic expectations

How Did We Get Here?

To discover where stress starts, we need to look at the typical development of a child. When we are born, none of us knows right from wrong; we have no concepts about what is good or bad; we do not expect things to be a certain way - we just experience life for what it is. As babies we are quite content as long as we are warm, fed, loved and without pain. As we grow, however, we naturally start to form concepts, opinions and ideas about what will make us happier, and these things depend on the environment that we are brought up in. In other words, a person brought up in New York City will have a very different set of values from someone raised on the west coast of Ireland. As we grow, we trustingly accept the values of those around us as our view of the world develops. If children are told a 'fact' at this impressionable age they will believe it without question. Misconceptions about life can therefore be handed down from generation to generation, and in this way we may form erroneous ideas or fixed prejudices which may remain with us throughout our lives.

Throughout childhood, teachers and parents, with every good intention, will try to influence us to live in the way that they think life should be lived. These ideas are often based on trying to give us the chances they wish they had had, and a genuine belief that they know what's best for us. Our whole education system is based on the assumption that if we pass examinations we will 'succeed' - that is, that the job and salary we get will give us happiness and make us feel important. Thus the conditioning to grin and bear our working life begins at school.

The Golden Cage

While listening to an educational programme on the radio recently, I heard a headmaster expressing his concern about the changes he saw in children during their school years. He saw children of five or six with bright eyes, smiling faces, beautiful posture and ease of movement; they were nearly always talkative, eager to please, willing to learn, had a playful nature and were generally enthusiastic about life. By the time these same children left school at 16 they hardly looked anyone in the eye, their posture was very slumped with rounded shoulders, they were often lazy and uncaring about the people around them and they generally looked unhappy. 'What,' this headmaster asked, 'in the name of education are we doing to our children to make them change so dramatically?'

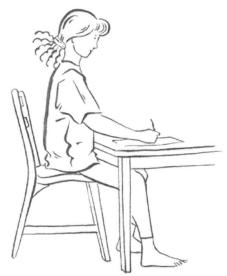

As children start their school life, they naturally have good posture

Perhaps all this comes about because for 11 years of our development we are placed in an institution full of 'must', 'have to', 'can't',

'should', 'got to' and 'ought to'. This has the detrimental effect of causing children gradually to lose their openness. They come to feel that
they must act in a way that fits in with the rest of society, and that if
they do not they will be ostracized by their peers. They have to learn
very quickly how to protect themselves from punishment and ridicule. As a result, many children become more introverted and will
often think that there is something wrong with them.

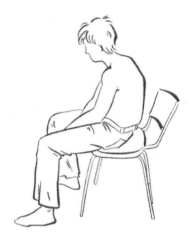

Teenager sitting slumped with rounded shoulders

British headmaster Michael Sullivan wrote in an article in the
Times Educational Supplement (18 October, 1985):

Self confidence is developed through the reduction of fear, stress,
uncertainty, confusion and failure - the very tools that too many
of us skilfully use in the management of children in our charge.
Children are fearful of verbal abuse, physical abuse and sarcasm.
Children are stressed on the rack of tests and quizzes, often facing
inevitable personal humiliation.

Many of us have endured similar traumas, but mostly we block out such memories because they are too painful to endure - yet our muscles remember them on an unconscious level. The protection that we acquire over those all-important years of our development manifests itself in muscle tension as our shoulders become rounded or hunched, our backs become arched and our stoops become more and more pronounced. These muscular tensions will subsequently affect the alignment of the rest of the body and can often be the seeds of future ill-health. They will affect our lives on every level unless we are willing to release them from our body. Child psychologists can often detect children who are emotionally disturbed simply by the way they hold their bodies or their breathing.

The Seat of the Problem

As soon as a child goes to school she is forced to sit in a chair, sometimes for long periods. The chair itself is very uncomfortable and not suited to her size or natural posture. The main reason for this is that the horizontal part of the chair, which takes most of the weight of the body, is *sloping backwards*.

The child, therefore, has no option but to tense many of her muscles to maintain her natural upright posture. Not liking the sense of 'falling backwards' that the chair produces, she will tilt forwards by raising her back legs off the floor. In this position the children can maintain her posture effortlessly.

The response from the teacher will be 'You might break the chair' or 'Someone could trip over the back legs' or 'You might tilt too far forwards and hurt yourself.' The damage to the child's posture is not even considered.

A child may then develop the technique of sitting on one leg, which also has the effect of raising up the pelvis, once again enabling her to maintain an upright posture. However, this is often actively discouraged as it can interfere with the flow of blood down the leg.

Children eventually become inured to sitting in backward sloping chairs for literally thousands and thousands of hours while at school. Sooner or later they begin to slump as their back muscles become more and more fatigued. To make the problem worse, the children then have to bend over their desks in order to read and write. Since it is impossible for them to use their hip joint efficiently, as the pelvis is already tilting backwards owing to the shape of the chair seat, they will then bend their spines, causing unnecessary wear and tear on the vertebrae and discs.

We ruin children's posture by making them sit on badly designed furniture and then, in our ignorance, criticize them for having poor posture. They are told to sit up straight and put their shoulders back; the only way to do this is to arch the lumber spine with more tension than ever. The children then begin to think that this is the way they *ought* to sit. Unfortunately, this posture becomes fixed within the body, often for the rest of our days, becoming progressively more painful as time goes on. (In fact, these days this problem may start even earlier than school, because most children's pushchairs and car seats also slope backwards.) It is hardly surprising that there are millions of people who suffer with pain in the lumbar region.

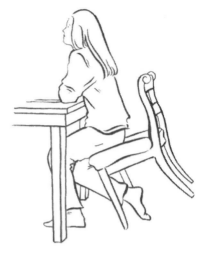

Girl tilting her chair forward in order to maintain good posture

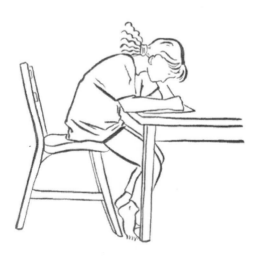

*Girl bending over her schoolwork - this is often
the cause of poor posture in later life*

Thinking to the Future

Even from the age of six or seven children are asked what they would like to be when they grow up, as if this were a decision that they really ought to be thinking about. From this time onwards children are geared towards goal-orientated examinations. Many people end up in jobs they dislike and have very little time left over in which to do what they really want. Feeling dissatisfied with their lot, they look towards promotion and more money to fulfil themselves. Of course, this satisfaction never comes as they are always looking for happiness in the future rather than in the present moment. Reshad Feild said once: 'If we are truly in the present moment, and are not being carried away by our thoughts and fantasies, then we are in a position to be free of fate and available to our destiny. When we are in the present moment, our work on Earth begins.'

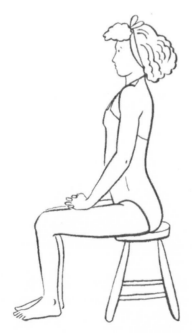

Girl 'sitting up straight' by arching her back

Stress at Home

The effects of the breakdown in the family structure have been confirmed by recent research showing that an increasing number of children are emotionally distressed. Many of these children feel frightened, lonely or depressed and can display symptoms such as nervousness, anxiety, inappropriate anger or unruly behaviour. As a result, both parents and teachers are witnessing more frequent instances of hostility aimed at themselves and other children.

In his book *Emotional Intelligence*, Daniel Goleman reports that according to recent surveys done in the US, Canada and New Zealand, as many as 20 per cent of children have severe psychological difficulties. Anxiety, ranging from general apprehension and constant worry to phobias which interfere with their daily lives, is the most common problem affecting children under the age of 11. These problems can then be responsible for the excessive consumption of alcohol during their teenage years. But perhaps the most disturbing development that we have seen in recent times is the increase in murder and violent crimes committed by children. In fact, in the US the number of murders committed by teenagers has quadrupled during the past 20 years.

Often, these deteriorating behaviour patterns are not dealt with, because parents and teachers are under considerable stress themselves and cannot always provide the time and support needed to cope constructively with their children's emotional demands. Some of these children will transfer their emotional problems to their future relationships as adults and will have little chance of enjoying a fulfilling and stable life. The story does not stop there; if, as is often the case, children's anxieties, worries and depressive behaviour are not dealt with in a loving and constructive way, they will pass on these aggressive and uncaring traits to their own offspring.

Families find themselves in a self-perpetuating cycle of stress and fear, with ever-worsening consequences. As the poem below suggests, the answer is incredibly simple, but to put these ideas into practice you have to set yourself against the nature of the world today:

If a child lives with criticism
He learns to condemn
If a child lives with hostility
He learns to fight
If a child lives with ridicule
He learns to be shy
If a child lives with shame
He learns to feel guilty
If a child lives with tolerance
He learns to be patient
If a child lives with encouragement
He learns confidence
If a child lives with praise
He learns to appreciate
If a child lives with fairness
He learns justice
If a child lives with security
He learns to have faith
If a child lives with approval
He learns to like himself
If a child lives with acceptance and friendship
He learns to find love in the world

Low Self-esteem

People with low self-esteem feel unable to say 'no' to the demands of others, even when they are already under great pressure themselves. They will often take on more than they can cope with and consequently buckle under the pressure. By un-learning the detrimental habits that have accumulated over the years, a person's self-confidence can increase and only then will he or she be able to gain more control over decision-making and avoiding taking on other people's problems. If this can be achieved, the person's mental and emotional health can greatly improve, causing other people to treat him or her with more respect. Time and time again I have seen that **those who accept only the best treatment in life will often receive it.** We all start out in life with high ideals, and it is only the inaccurate concepts and beliefs that have been imposed on us that mould us into what we have become. We need to separate our true selves from the false persona that we adopt.

This is exactly what the Alexander Technique can help us to achieve. It can help us to rid ourselves of the physical tensions which have been built up since childhood, and of the mental and emotional strains which often accompany them.

An Antidote to Stress

Many of us have forgotten how to relax and enjoy life, and this we must do if we are ever to have a chance of being truly happy. When we are under stress we can no longer think clearly or objectively, because we react subconsciously to all the stimuli to which we are subjected. We need to realize that, although we have been taught to seek happiness constantly in our worldly activities, true contentment is closer to us than our own breath. The joy of owning a new house or car, having a new job or relationship, getting married or even having a baby can so often be short lived. And the very same things that brought us so much happiness often turn out to be the biggest causes of stress in our lives - the burden of paying the mortgage, the first scratch on the bodywork, pressures at work, marital arguments, or the infant who keeps us up all night. What is so surprising is that many of us continue to think that all these things will eventually make us happy, so we make the same errors time and time again without becoming any wiser. Alexander summed this up by changing the well-known motto: 'If at first you don't succeed, try, try again' to 'If at first you don't succeed, never try again - at least not in the same way!'

The first step towards living a more fulfilling life is to begin to understand what really makes us happy. It may be that we need to re-define our idea about success and failure, as did Ralph Waldo Emerson (in his work, *Self-reliance and Other Essays*):

> *To laugh often and love much, to win the respect of intelligent persons and the affection of children; to earn the approbation of honest critics and to endure the betrayal of false friends; to appreciate beauty; to find the best in others; to give one's self; to leave the world a bit better, whether by a healthy child, a garden patch or a redeemed social condition; to have played and laughed with enthusiasm and sung with exultation; to know even one life has breathed easier because you have lived, this is to have succeeded.*

Yet the irony is that if we become stressed in our efforts to obtain happiness we can acquire the habit of being tense, which will persist for the rest of our lives, leading to ill-health. Stress often starts in the mind, yet is immediately transmitted to the body.

The second step is to realize that we have become programmed to look for our happiness, peace and contentment in future goals - but this is not where these gifts lie. We need to re-programme ourselves to start seeing life in a new way.

This change is difficult because most of our reactions are subconscious: we are simply not aware which of them are no longer appropriate. We become so accustomed to behaving in certain ways that the only way to get through the maze of unconscious behaviour is to use a mirror: the Alexander Technique acts as just that.

The Origins of the Technique

Alexander developed his Technique in response to his own severe speech problem. An Australian actor and orator who lived from 1869 to 1955, his livelihood and vocation were threatened by these health problems, and the search for a solution led Alexander to various discoveries about the body and its interrelationship with the mind and emotions. These discoveries were the signposts on his long journey of self-discovery, which brought about not only the answer to his particular ailments, but to the development of a new philosophy for living.

Alexander became aware during this process that not just individuals but the entire planet was being harmed by the way we live. He could see that greed and selfishness cause many people to be so goal-orientated (what he termed 'end-gaining') that we do not stop to consider the consequences of their actions.

'End-gaining'

In his book *Constructive Conscious Control of the Individual*, Alexander spoke of his conviction that, while we are frequently told that the cause of our difficulties is the increasing complexity of life, our real dilemma stems from the way in which we cultivate within ourselves a condition of stress and strain (which in our ignorance we look upon as something apart from ourselves) in an effort to adapt to our ever-changing environment.

For Alexander a singular example of this self-imposed stress was the phenomenon of always looking to the future, instead of in the present moment, for self-validation and happiness. A clear instance of this is many people's experience of Christmas. For a number of weeks preceding the holiday, preparations are made and people spend a great deal of time, money and energy to ensure that their celebrations will be enjoyable. At last Christmas Day arrives and everything is in place - there is nothing left to do except enjoy the festivities. But what do we encounter? A barrage of advertisements on the telly enticing us to exotic, far-off holiday destinations, or to the nearby shopping centre where the sales are about to begin. Before Christmas day is even halfway through begin to wander yet again from the present moment to future desires. This is an example of what Alexander called *end-gaining* behaviour in action, and it is a common source of stress.

Freedom of Choice

Alexander talked at length about freedom of choice; it is fundamental to his Technique. He realized that many people would perceive his Technique as a method of performing actions in certain ways, yet he was adamant that it was nothing of the kind, but instead a way of reclaiming free choice. If you examine people under stress, you will find that they feel trapped in a situation they are unable to do anything about, and they will often use one of the following words or phrases to describe their plight:

must	should	shouldn't	got to
ought to	ought not	have to	can't

These words are disempowering. Freedom of choice is so important to us that many millions of people have died in countless wars trying to preserve this precious right, yet today it is being subtly eroded. We think we are free because we live in a 'free country', but in reality how many of us really *feel* free? Just listen to a person who is stressed and you will probably hear one of these phrases:

- I *should* be at work on time.
- I *must* go now because otherwise I am going to be late.
- I *have* got to finish this work before tomorrow.
- I *can't* get to my appointment because of the traffic.
- I *have* to cook the meals every day.
- I *ought* to go and do the housework.

If you are under stress at the moment, it might be useful to consider how often you use this type of phraseology when describing your situation.

The word stress itself indicates that one part of an object is going one way as another part is going in the opposite direction; in fact, the dictionary definition of stress is *to be drawn tight by a system of forces*. A piece of string or a bridge, say, can be stressed when there are two forces acting on it in different directions, but what are the opposing forces that are acting on us when we feel stressed? *The desire to do what is enjoyable and the feeling of obligation to do what we think we 'ought' to be doing.* Stress occurs when we don't even see that we have this much of a choice, feeling instead that we must always fulfil our obligations whatever the personal cost.

The Alexander Technique involves making decisions during all of your actions, and by doing so will come to realize that you have a much wider variety of choices than you thought. By exercising this choice during your physical movements, you will learn that you can apply the same principles to your mental and emotional reactions. Alexander saw his Technique as a way of giving us the opportunity to choose to react in a different way - a way that does not produce stress in the first place, a method whose true purpose is to restore real freedom of choice to each and every human being. Any stress-reduction technique that does not change our reaction to external stimuli by altering the way in which we think and react will be merely cosmetic and will therefore bring only temporary relief.

The Alexander Technique is not merely a physical technique that can help to improve posture and movement, but deals with every issue that mankind faces today. Reason, choice and common sense are vital qualities which we have all been given, but we are not really taught how to utilize them to our greatest advantage. Many of us just do as everyone else does. To stand up for what you know to be true against tremendous external pressures does take a great deal of courage, but unless we do so we will never really feel satisfied.

Happiness

Alexander was convinced that in the human endeavour to become happier, most people were actually achieving the opposite.

He felt that the majority of adults were 'experiencing a continual deterioration of their psycho-physical selves' due to the fact that there were so many stimuli causing people irritation and internal pressure both night and day. In *Constructive Conscious Control of the Individual*, Alexander wrote that under these conditions it should come as no surprise that people are unhappy. Irritation is not compatible with happiness, yet any efforts to fight off the irritation will only increase a person's aggravation and diminish his or her chances of long-term happiness.

Hint

The Alexander Technique is the tool which shows us how to be free through awareness and conscious control of our thoughts, enabling us safely and effectively to restore equilibrium to our lives. Practising the Technique is a process of un-learning detrimental habits which can enable us to rediscover our true essence.

The principles and concepts of the Alexander Technique described in Chapter 2 can help you to examine your life and to make the necessary changes that will assist you to live in a more harmonious way. This can help with individual health problems and can also lead to greater awareness of the consequences of our actions on others and on our environment.

2
Principles of the Alexander Technique

We learn wisdom from failure much more than from success; we often discover what will do, by finding out what will not do; and probably he who never made a mistake never made a discovery.

Samuel Smiles

The pace of life seems to increase each year and many people are finding it more and more difficult to cope with the stresses that our hurried way of life brings about. Recently there has been a trend of 'downshifting' as people move to less stressful environments, choose to have fewer material possessions, or generally simplify their lives. While this is obviously a step in the right direction, not everyone is in the privileged position of being able to make these changes, and even if you can 'downshift' you are still likely to be holding tension within yourself habitually without realizing it. Even if you do not want to change your job or lifestyle, you can still 'de-stress' yourself by practising the Alexander Technique.

Stress and the Alexander Technique

Many people know that the Alexander Technique can improve posture or help those who suffer from back, neck or shoulder problems. Although the Technique can be very useful in these areas, it can also be invaluable when applied to many other aspects of life, such as during pregnancy and early motherhood, improving self-confidence, or while playing sport or music. What many people do not realize is that the Alexander Technique can also be extremely effective in combating the effects of stress which, as we have seen, are among the most common health problems in society today. The Technique can do this by making you more conscious of yourself and situations in which you are likely to encounter stress; it can help you to reduce stress levels in both your body and mind. It can have a profound effect on your mental and emotional well-being, and people who practise the Technique often report feeling happier in themselves and more at ease with others. As the stress level in your body drops, you will find that you are more able to cope with everyday problems as they arise. The amount of conflict, both internal and external, is often reduced, allowing a more peaceful and harmonious way of living.

Alexander's personal journey of self-discovery, which is described in detail later in this chapter, not only freed him from the causes of stress, but led him to a place where he could help others to escape from their mental and emotional turmoil. This book will help you to understand the principles and concepts that he discovered, and will allow you to embark on a similar journey of your own. To get to the same place as he did we must travel on the same route; unlike Alexander, however, we do have a map and directions.

Tip

It is important to realize that if you care for your body and mind now they will serve you better later on.

Personal Education

Although the Alexander Technique has far-reaching effects, it is at the same time simple and easy to follow, but you will need patience and a willingness to take responsibility for yourself. By progressively becoming aware and letting go of physical and mental tension, you will be able to achieve a more relaxed muscular system and a calmer mind. This can then relieve or prevent many psycho-physical illnesses by enabling your body to function more freely. Since the way in which you move or hold yourself affects your mental and emotional outlook on life, releasing muscular tension will help you to become calmer and happier. In short, the Alexander Technique can help you to lead a more enjoyable life, because if the body is less stressed and the mind less anxious you will experience life in a completely different way.

As we have seen, Alexander developed his Technique not only as a way of improving posture and physical health, but as a way of freeing humanity from its 'fixed prejudices' and 'erroneous concepts'. His Technique is based on the premise that there is an inseparable unity between the body, mind and emotions, and he firmly believed that mental stress leads to muscle tension and eventually to emotional instability. He saw his Technique as a journey of self-discovery and hoped that his experience might "one day be recognized as a signpost directing the explorer to a country hitherto 'undiscovered', and one which offers unlimited opportunity for fruitful research to the patient and observant pioneer."

A number of famous writers and philosophers, including Aldous Huxley, George Bernard Shaw and Professor John Dewey, had personal contact with Alexander and realized the importance of the philosophy and practical experience behind his Technique. Their writings often reflected the principles and ideas behind the Technique; Aldous Huxley claimed that a student of the Alexander Technique "can often change his entire attitude to life and cure his neurotic tendencies". George Bernard Shaw claimed that "Alexander established not only the beginnings of a far reaching science of the apparently involuntary movements we call reflexes, but a technique of correction and self control which forms a substantial addition to our very slender resources in personal education." John Dewey said that Alexander's discovery "contains in my judgement the promise and potentiality of the new direction that is needed in all education".

The famous philosopher Plato once said that a life unexamined is not worth living. How often do we really think things through and try to make some sense of our existence? The Alexander Technique is one of the best tools I know for helping us to analyse this human existence.

History of the Technique

Frederick Matthias Alexander was born on 20th January 1869 in a small town called Wynyard, situated on the northwest coast of Tasmania. From birth he was a very weak child, suffering from asthma and other respiratory illnesses throughout his childhood. Due to his frail health, he was taken out of school at an early age. During the day he would help look after his father's horses; in the evenings he would be taught at home by the local school teacher. The sensitivity of touch which he developed in his hands may well have originated while handling the horses.

As Alexander got older, his health gradually improved. By the time he was 17, financial pressures on the family had forced him to leave the outdoor life which he loved so much and go out to work. When not at work, Alexander took part in amateur dramatics and taught himself to play the violin. By the age of 20 he had saved up enough money to travel to Melbourne, where he stayed with an uncle. For the next three months his uncle took him to the theatre, concerts and art galleries, and by the end of his stay Alexander had resolutely decided to train as an actor and reciter.

Voice Problems

Alexander stayed in Melbourne to undertake his training, and it was not long before he gained a reputation as a first-class reciter and went on to form his own theatre company specializing in Shakespearean recitals. As he became increasingly successful, Alexander began to accept more and more engagements. He also had to perform in front of larger and larger audiences in big venues where, since he did not use a microphone, he had to project his own voice quite far. This put more and more strain on his vocal cords, and within a short time the stress began to show - his voice regularly became hoarse in the middle of his performances, and on occasion Alexander lost his voice completely.

> It is important to realize that although Alexander's problems revolved in the first instance around his voice, the principles of the Technique are relevant to any stress-related condition.

Medical Investigations

Alexander became desperate, not only because his career was in jeopardy but because his happiness revolved so much around the theatre. Everything he had grown to love was now being threatened. He approached various doctors and voice trainers who gave him medication and exercises to perform, but nothing seemed to make any difference. The situation deteriorated until on one occasion Alexander could barely finish a recital. He became more and more worried as he realized that there might not be a solution to his curious problem. He approached another doctor, one of the leading throat specialists in Australia at that time. After this doctor had examined Alexander he was convinced that the vocal cords had merely been over-strained; he then prescribed complete rest for Alexander's voice for two weeks and promised that this would cure his ailment. Determined to try anything, Alexander uttered hardly uttered a word over the next fortnight.

When he began his first recital after this period he was delighted to find that his voice was crystal clear; better, in fact, than it had been for a long time. But, to his dismay, after only a short while into the recital the hoarseness in his voice returned. By the end of the evening he could hardly speak. Feeling very disillusioned, Alexander returned to the doctor and reported what had happened. The doctor, however, was optimistic and felt that his treatment had been effective, if only for a short time. He advised Alexander to continue the treatment, but this time he prescribed vocal rest for a further month.

Self-discovery

Alexander decided that he would not follow the doctor's advice this time. If two weeks' rest had only given him about an hour's cure, what would be the point of remaining virtually silent for another month? He could not spend his life not talking, and he argued with the doctor that if his voice was in perfect condition when he started the recital, yet in an appalling state by the time he had finished, it must have been *something that he was doing while performing* that was causing the hoarseness. Although the doctor agreed that this must be the case, he had no idea as to what that 'something' was.

Alexander left the surgery determined to find the cause of his peculiar problem himself. His ensuing journey of self-discovery eventually provided him not only with the answer to his dilemma, but to the evolution of a new philosophy for living. At the same time He also unearthed a cause and contributory factor of humanity's mental, emotional and physical suffering.

Alexander's findings have been greatly underestimated and still today many people are ignorant of their full potential; his discovery may yet turn out to be one of the greatest of the 20th century.

Unconscious Habits

Alexander started his investigations with just one clue to follow up: when he recited his voice became hoarse, but when he spoke in his normal manner the hoarseness disappeared. Following a few logical steps, Alexander deduced that since ordinary speaking did not cause him to lose his voice, while reciting did, there must be something different about what he did when reciting. If he could find out what that difference was, he might be able to change the way in which he was using his voice when reciting, which would then solve his problem.

He used a mirror to observe himself carefully when he was speaking in his normal voice and then again when reciting, in the hope that he could discern some difference between the two. He watched carefully, and noticed three differences:

1. *While reciting, he would forcibly pull his head back and down on to his spine.*

2. *He simultaneously depressed his larynx (the cavity in the throat where the vocal cords are situated).*

3. *He also sucked air in through his mouth, producing a gasping sound.*

Up to this point Alexander had been completely unaware that he had developed these three habits, and when he returned to his normal speaking voice he realized that the same tendencies were also present but to a much smaller degree, which was why they had previously gone undetected and presumably why they had done less harm. Thus he formulated his first discovery:

Misuse of the body often occurs habitually and unconsciously.

Alexander returned to the mirror, encouraged that he was close to solving his problem, and began to recite over and over again to see if he could discover any more information that might help him. He soon noticed that the three tendencies became more accentuated when he was reading a difficult passage that placed unusual demands on his voice. This confirmed his earlier suspicion that there was a definite connection between the way in which he recited and the hoarseness. For the first time he realized that he was unconsciously causing his own problem.

Cause and Effect

To further his exploration, Alexander then had to work out what was responsible for these tendencies. Was it the sucking in of air that caused the pulling back of the head and the depressing of the larynx? Or was it the pulling back of the head that caused the depressing of the larynx and the sucking in of the air? Or was it the depressing of the larynx that caused the other two? After much experimentation, he realized that he could not directly prevent the sucking in of air or the depression of the larynx, but he could to some extent prevent pulling his head back, by releasing muscle tension. When he did not pull his head back as much, he noticed that the state of the larynx improved and he did not suck in air while breathing. This consequently decreased the hoarseness in his voice, thereby proving that his ingrained habit of over-tensing his neck muscles, which resulted in him pulling his head back, was at the root of his problem. At this point in his experimentation he wrote in his own personal account:

> *The importance of this discovery cannot be overestimated, for through it I was lead on to the further discovery of the Primary Control of the workings of all the mechanisms of the human organism, and this marked the first important stage of my investigation.*

The Primary Control

Throughout the body are located a series of mechanisms of postural reflexes which constantly reassess our balance. Their function is to provide us with fluidity or grace of movement as we go about our everyday movements. The Primary Control is the name Alexander gave to the dynamic relationship between the head, neck and back which he found governs the workings of all these mechanisms and reflexes. In order to function efficiently, it is crucial that this relationship is not interfered with by muscular tension. Any fixed position of the head or neck, even if straight, will invariably interfere with its function. If freedom of movement is to be attained it is essential that the Primary Control is allowed to work without restriction. Thus Alexander's second discovery:

The way in which the body is used will invariably affect all of its various functions.

To obtain proof of his theory, Alexander returned to his doctor, and after further examination it was confirmed that there had been a considerable improvement in the general condition of his throat and vocal cords. He was now convinced beyond a shadow of a doubt that the way in which he was reciting was causing him to lose his voice, and that changing the way in which he performed would eventually make his voice strong and healthy again. However, Alexander was still left with the question of why was he pulling back his head in the first place.

Faulty Sensory Perception

Excited by the idea that he was getting to the bottom of the matter, Alexander experimented with different head and neck positions to see if he could improve his voice even further. During one of these experiments he deliberately put his head forward, hoping for an improvement, but was amazed to find that this had the opposite effect, again depressing the larynx. To have a closer look at how he was moving from different angles, he added two further mirrors on either side of the original one. When he observed himself in these mirrors he could see clearly that although he had intended to put his head in a forward direction, he was actually still pulling his head back and down on to his spine as before. Alexander was amazed at these findings, because he realized that even though he'd felt that he was putting his head forwards, he could see with his own eyes that he was not. He had just discovered the third, and one of the most important, principles behind his Technique:

The existence of faulty sensory perception.

In other words, Alexander could no longer rely on his sensory feelings to tell him where his body was in space or even what he was or was not doing with different parts of his body. At first he thought this was his own personal idiosyncrasy, but when, at a later date, he started to teach his Technique to other people he realized that nearly everyone suffers from similar delusions and that faulty sensory perception is very common.

When beginning, many Alexander students will swear that they are, for example holding their head straight when it is, in fact, on one side. As a result, their balance and co-ordination are adversely affected and they may even be in pain. When the teacher gently straightens their head it will feel to them at first as though their head is now crooked to one side, and they won't be convinced until they can see for themselves in a mirror. This is one reason why the Technique cannot be learned from books alone; you need help from an Alexander teacher who will be able to give you direct feedback about what you are doing with your body at any given time.

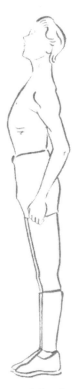

This man is convinced that he is standing up
straight when he is clearly 'bow' shaped

Alexander used to say that everyone wants to be right, but
hardly anyone stops for a moment to consider if their idea
of right is really right. He therefore advised his pupils to pre-
sume that they were wrong to start with.

Holistic Discovery

Alexander, like most of us, had relied on his sensory perceptions to
give him information about his body and surroundings. Now he was
felt he had reached an enormous setback. How could he now bring

about the release of tension in his neck muscles? He also began to realize that his habit of pulling his head back was not only causing the depression of his larynx, but also many tensions and stresses throughout his entire body. He was lifting his chest, arching his back, throwing his pelvis forward, over-tightening his leg muscles and even gripping the floor with his feet. This was affecting his entire balance and posture. These revelations led to his fourth discovery:

> *Parts of the body do not function as separate entities, but work as a whole unit with each part affecting all the other parts.*

Stimuli And Reactions

During his training to be an actor, Alexander had been taught by one of his recital tutors to 'take hold of the floor' with his feet. He had complied with his tutor's instructions by tensing his feet and toes and actually trying to grip the floor. At the time he had dutifully followed his teacher's instructions without question. Now, however, Alexander realized that tightening the muscles in his legs and feet was part of the same habit causing him to tighten his neck muscles. The action of 'taking hold of the floor' with his feet had over the years become such an ingrained habit that he was completely unaware that he was doing it. He found it extremely difficult to recite without all his old accompanying physical habits, and his first attempts at changing them simply increased his muscle tension. Thus his fifth discovery:

> *A given stimulus produces the same reaction over and over again which, if it goes unchecked, turns into habitual*

behaviour and will eventually feel normal and natural to us, no matter how detrimental this habit is to our health.

This last principle is very useful in understanding how stress builds up, since tension during our daily activities can feel totally normal and can be repeated again and again over many years.

Changing the Pattern of Thought

Alexander then started to think about how he consciously used his body while reciting, and had to admit to himself that he gave little thought to how he moved, but simply acted in a way that was habitual because this felt 'right' to him. At first he performed conscious actions such as putting his head forward and up, but found that this once again increased the muscular tension he was trying to eliminate. At this point he gave up in exasperation, and in doing so achieved the release of tension he had wanted for so long. Alexander realized that he merely had to change the way he *thought* in order to produce a corresponding change in the muscle tension that had been at the root of his problem. He began to construct a system of 'Directions' which would directly release his muscular tension. Alexander described a 'Direction' as:

A process which involves projecting messages from the brain to the body's mechanisms, and conducting the energy necessary for the use of these mechanisms.

There are two kinds of Directions, referred to as 'Primary Directions' and 'Secondary Directions'.

Primary Directions

Most of the problems which stem from poor posture can be traced to over-tensed neck muscles which interfere with the freedom of the head in relationship to the neck and spine. If this relationship is interfered with it will be impossible to obtain any lasting freedom of movement elsewhere in the body.

The Primary Directions are:

- Allow there to be freedom of your neck.
- Allow your head to go forward and up.
- Allow your back to lengthen and widen.

It is important that these Primary Directions are followed in sequence, as it is impossible to allow your head to go forward and up if you have not released the tension in your neck; likewise, it is impossible to achieve the beneficial lengthening of the spine if your head is not going forward and up.

Allow There to Be Freedom of Your Neck

The pivot point of the head is located at the top of spine, much higher than many people at first realize. The centre of gravity of the head is situated forward of the pivot point, which means that the head is naturally inclined to move in a forward direction. The purpose of this Direction is to release the excessive tension that often exists in this area, which causes the head to be pulled back and down on to the spine, thus interfering with the natural balance of the head. It is important to realize that neck tension may be difficult to detect, because often we have become used to the feeling over a long period of time.

Allow Your Head to Go Forward and Up

You should think of your head going in a direction that is forward and up *in relation to your spine*, not in relation to your environment. Body mechanisms are arranged in such a way that the head leads a movement and the body follows. Allowing the head to go forward helps this natural organization to occur, allowing all our movements to be performed with the greatest efficiency.

Allow Your Back to Lengthen and Widen

This Direction will help you to reduce tension throughout the upper part of your body. Expanding this area will improve your breathing and allow the internal organs more space, enabling them to function more efficiently. It will also prevent a shortening of the spine, which can cause or aggravate back and neck pain. Releasing tension in the upper part of your body will also ease the downward pressure which causes unnecessary restriction in the hips, legs and feet and makes standing and walking more difficult. By thinking of your back lengthening and widening, your spine will be encouraged to elongate rather than shorten, and this is often accompanied by a feeling of lightness and ease.

Secondary Directions

Secondary Directions can be used as a supplement to the Primary Directions to release tension in localized parts of your body. Unlike the Primary Directions, they do not necessarily directly affect the functioning of the Primary Control. Some common Secondary Directions which can be useful in reducing levels of stress are:

- *Allow your shoulders to release away from one another.* This will help anyone with rounded shoulders or who has shallow breathing or asthma.

- *Allow your left shoulder to release away from your right hip, and your right shoulder to release away from your left hip.* As we have seen, leaning over a school or office desk for many years can often cause a slumped posture. This Direction can be very helpful in releasing the tension that is responsible for this.

- *Imagine your fingers lengthening as the palm of your hand widens.* This can help anyone who unconsciously clenches their fists when under stress.

- *Think of allowing your to jaw drop away from your ears.* This will help to release tension in the jaw muscle, which is common to those under stress.

- *Think of not pushing your pelvis forward.* This can prevent an over-arching of the back, which is a common habit of those who suffer with back pain.

- *Think of not bracing your knees back.* This can be effective in releasing tension in the legs, which again is common in those who have poor posture.

- *Think of your feet spreading on to the ground as your toes lengthen.* This can release tension in the toes and will help you to stand and walk more with more poise.

These are just a few examples of the many Secondary Directions. Breathing awareness (see Chapter 8) may also be of benefit.

Whichever Direction is followed, it always involves *thinking* of one part of your body moving away from another part, allowing a lengthening and widening of your entire being. This is in contrast to muscle tension, which by its very nature causes the muscles concerned to shorten in length - the phenomenon behind Alexander's sixth discovery:

Mind, body and emotions are inseparable and therefore have a direct effect upon each another.

Goal Orientation

Alexander practised thinking of his Directions long and hard, yet when he returned to the mirrors he found that he failed to put them into practice far more often than he succeeded. However, he was sure that he was very close to succeeding, and searched for the possible causes of his failure. After many months he saw that he was able to give his Directions successfully right up to the moment of reciting, but then would revert back to his old habits.

He had to find a way of stopping his harmful habits. At this point he came up with his seventh discovery:

Being too goal-orientated can prevent you from achieving your objective.

Inhibition

Alexander realized that the only way he could prevent his old habits from resurfacing was to *inhibit any immediate response* to the stimulus of, in his case, speaking a sentence, and to keep on inhibiting while he was performing his task. Inhibition is the fundamental key behind the Alexander Technique, for without it we do not have a chance to give the *Directions* nor can we change the way in which we react to situations. It was not easy for Alexander to inhibit a response that had become so familiar over the years, yet this very response, which *felt so right and natural* to him, was at the root of his problem, and therefore had to be replaced by a different way of being that *felt alien and even wrong.*

In recent times the word *inhibition* has come to mean the suppression of feelings or the inability to be spontaneous, but this is mainly because the famous psychologist Sigmund Freud used the term in this particular context. The dictionary definition of inhibition is: *The restraint of direct expression of an instinct.* If this restraint stems from fear and is unconscious, then it could be seen as involving an unhealthy form of suppression and therefore have a negative connotation. However, Alexander used the term to mean deliberate restraint in order to make a more conscious decision, which can have very beneficial results. Dr Jacob Bronowski, author of The Ascent of Man, went so far as to say: "'We are nature's unique experiment to make the rational intelligence prove sounder than the reflex. Success or failure of this experiment depends on the basic human ability to impose a delay between the stimulus and the response.'" This states exactly what Alexander meant. In his book *Body Awareness in Action* Professor Frank Pierce Jones describes inhibition as 'the fundamental process, conscious or unconscious, by which the integrity of the organism is maintained while a particular response is being carried out, or not carried out, as the case may be. It is the failure of inhibition that more than anything else is responsible for the dangerous state of the world. Restoring inhibition so that it can perform its integrative function on a conscious level should be the primary aim of education.'

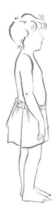

Unlike many adults, children naturally inhibit before moving

Through the process of stopping and consciously choosing a different way of reacting, Alexander gained great control over his habits. It helped him to prevent the automatic reactions which had been at the root of his vocal problem. A moment's pause gave him the opportunity to refrain from pulling his head back, depressing his larynx and sucking in air at the vital moment of speaking.

Winston Churchill once said that men stumble over the truth from time to time, but most of them pick themselves up and hurry on as though nothing had happened. Alexander did indeed stumble on an amazing discovery and we are extremely fortunate today that he did not pick himself up and pretend that nothing had happened!

Teaching the Technique

When, finally, Alexander was able to prevent his habitual responses, not only was he freed from the voice problem which had jeopardized his career, but he also cured himself of the recurring asthma that had afflicted him from infancy. Alexander returned to the stage to continue his career as an actor. Many of his colleagues sought his help with their performance problems, and he began teaching his Technique to them. News of Alexander's successes spread quickly and doctors began referring some of their patients to him.

Using the gentle guidance of his hands as well as verbal instructions to convey the principles of his Technique, Alexander helped many people to overcome the harmful habits which were at the root of their various ailments. In the spring of 1904, he travelled to London in order to bring his Technique to a wider audience. He set up a practice in Victoria Street and later at Ashley Place in central London, and worked there until his death in October 1955.

During his life he attracted a great deal of interest from scientists and medical doctors, but was unable during his lifetime to substantiate his discoveries with scientific proof. This was partly because he was very protective of his Technique and reluctant to put it into the hands of scientists, whom, he felt, might distort his findings. In addition it is only recently that medical researchers have had the inclination or resources to research how we react mentally and emotionally to our environment. Although there is a long way to go before the true value of the Alexander Technique is recognized, more and more research and anecdotal evidence points to the fact that the Technique offers a positive and beneficial alternative way of dealing with many health problems.

Principles behind the Alexander Technique

- The body does not function as a number of separate entities, but works as one unit with each part affecting every other part.

- The mind, body and emotions are inseparable and in so being have a direct effect on one another.

- The way we use ourselves will invariably affect the various functions of the body and mind.

- The misuse of ourselves often occurs habitually and unconsciously.

- A given stimulus produces the same reaction over and over again, which, if unchecked, can turn into habitual behaviour; these habits will eventually feel normal and natural to us no matter how detrimental they are to our health.

- Most people suffer from faulty sensory perception; in other words, they cannot accurately determine the true position or movements of their body.

- Many erroneous preconceived ideas and fixed prejudices, which have their origins in childhood, continue to exert control over our adult selves.

- A goal-orientated or 'end-gaining' attitude can prevent people from achieving their objective and often causes tension, stress and pain.

- The Alexander Technique involves a process of re-educating the whole person.

- The Alexander Technique is a process of un-learning physical, mental and emotional habits and replacing them with conscious control of actions, thoughts and feelings.

  Putting the Alexander Technique into practice:

1. *Practise Inhibition.*

2. *Remain conscious of your thoughts and actions.*

3. *Use your thoughts alone to bring about a change where necessary.*

4. Exhibit free choice in thought, emotions and action.

3
The Physical
Effects of
Stress

The true miracle is not to fly in the air, or to walk on water ... but to walk on this earth.

Chinese Proverb

Alexander once said that we translate everything physical, mental or spiritual into muscular tension, and that therefore the mental stress we experience can affect our physical body in a variety of ways. These physical effects are often more noticeable to others than to ourselves. If this inappropriate muscle tension persists over a long period of time, it can affect every other system in the body.

Muscle accounts for approximately half our body weight, and therefore over-tense muscles can have a devastating effect on all our internal functions as well as on our posture and how we move. If we are suffering from stress we will be less likely to notice this muscle tension build-up until we find ourselves afflicted with a 'sudden' illness. We are so busy trying to cope with the pressures of life we give ourselves little time to be aware of our physical feelings. Our body gives us plenty of warning that things are not as they should be, but we usually either ignore the signs or are completely oblivious to them. You often hear people say that they 'don't have time to be ill', but if we push ourselves to the limits we must expect the consequences. The common warning sign is pain, and the effects of excessive muscle tension can be seen in the millions of people who suffer with backache, shoulder tension, migraines and headaches. Once we are in pain the body tenses up even more, and many people find themselves in a vicious circle which can, at best, be only temporarily relieved by medical treatment.

Infectious Diseases

Stress can also be partly responsible for the many infectious diseases from which we suffer, such as colds or flu. We are continually exposed to these viruses, but under normal circumstances our body has the ability to combat their effects. While under stress, however, the immune system starts to become less efficient because we are drained of energy. During recent investigations by psychologist Sheldon Cohen, working with scientists at a specialized colds research unit in Sheffield, England, two groups of subjects were exposed to the common cold virus: one group was made up of people suffering from stress, the other from those who weren't. It was found that nearly half the people who were under stress caught the cold, compared with only 27 per cent of those who were not under pressure.

Deadly Diseases

Extensive research has also been carried out by Bruce McEwen, a psychologist at Yale University in the US, who found that stress reduces the effectiveness of the immune system. He found that stress can increase vulnerability to viral infections, speed up the spread of cancer cells through the body, exacerbate asthma, cause a build-up of plaque in the circulation leading to blood clotting, speed up the onset of diabetes, lead to digestive problems such as duodenal and stomach ulcers, and even cause heart problems. It is therefore becoming increasingly clear that if we don't address the problem of stress we may not only be living unhappy lives, but unnecessarily brief ones.

The Alexander Technique has helped people to overcome a wide range of physical problems, including:

Pain with Muscle or Joint Problems

- Backache
- Neckache
- Headache
- Migraine
- Arthritis
- Repetitive Strain Injury (RSI)

Blood Circulation or Heart Problems

- High blood pressure
- Poor circulation
- Coronary thrombosis

Respiratory Problems

- Asthma
- Shallow breathing
- Hyperventilation

Digestive Problems

- Ulcers
- Heartburn

- Constipation
- Indigestion

Nervous Problems

- Trapped nerves
- Overactive nervous system
- Clumsiness

While the majority of people start to have Alexander lessons because of pain or illness, it is important to realize that you do not have to have something wrong with you to benefit from learning and applying the Alexander Technique. Some people come for lessons to improve their posture or because they lack confidence, while others come as a preventative measure so that they can avoid health problems now and later in life.

Symptoms of Stress

It is important to detect stress as early as possible. Prolonged exposure to any stressful situation may cause one of the following physical symptoms:

- fatigue
- headaches
- dizziness or even fainting
- breathlessness
- heart palpitations
- increased perspiration
- trembling of hands
- loss of sex drive
- change in sleep patterns
- digestive problems (in extreme cases nausea or vomiting may occur)
- increased physical sensitivity

There are other mental and emotional symptoms which often accompany the physical symptoms, and these will be dealt with in later chapters.

Fight or Flight

Stress and panic are normal reactions to danger - they are our natural response to fear. It is natural to become stressed if you are confronted by a ferocious dog or become separated from your child in a large crowd of people. These two situations are potentially life-threatening and the panic you experience is the body's pre-programmed way of reacting to the possible dangers that may arise. During this reaction, specific physiological changes take place: the adrenal glands become more active; the heart rate increases, the breathing becomes more rapid; the entire muscular system becomes tense; the pupils dilate and the level of sugar in the blood increases. These changes make us more alert and ready to cope with the emergency at hand. When the danger has passed, our body's functions gradually return to normal. This reaction is sometimes called the 'fight or flight' response; it provides the body with the necessary strength, speed and stamina for survival. We are well equipped to cope with the changes that the body undergoes as long as the situation is short-lived, but we are not, it seems, designed to cope with frequent fearful experiences over a long period of time.

In the 1930s an American doctor, Hans Selye, was one of the first people to analyse in depth the human response to severe stress. He described the body's adjustment to prolonged stress as the 'General Adaptation Syndrome', and divided the stress response into three phases:

1. The Alarm Response

2. Adaptation

3. Exhaustion

The Alarm Response

The Alarm Response is the immediate reaction to the impending danger. This response is controlled by the endocrine system, which regulates various bodily functions including the immune system, metabolism, respiration, sex hormones and allergic responses. Stressful situations activate the endocrine glands, which include the adrenal, pituitary and hypothalamus; these then secrete hormones into the bloodstream. These hormones, adrenalin, noradrenalin, cortisol, testosterone and thyroxine, are powerful stimulants and produce the following responses:

- increased heart rate

- increased blood pressure

- increased blood sugar, fats and cholesterol

- increased breathing rate

- increased muscle tension

- mental alertness

These responses prepare you to cope with the emergency at hand.

Adaptation

If any stressful situation is prolonged, then the body adapts accordingly. This stage is not necessarily harmful, *providing* the person has periods of rest and relaxation to counterbalance the tension caused during the stress response. During this stage, people may be prone to lapses in concentration, irritability, lethargy, physical tiredness and mental fatigue.

Exhaustion

If the stress continues over a long period, the body can no longer cope and the person will experience 'burn out'. They will suffer from adrenal exhaustion, which occurs when blood sugar levels decrease as the adrenalin supply becomes depleted. This leads to a dramatic reduction in the person's tolerance to stressful situations and soon they will be physically, mentally and emotionally exhausted. If nothing is done to redress the balance, the person will eventually become ill or even collapse.

Reducing Stress Levels

The first step in reducing the level of stress in our body is to understand exactly what happens to us when we become stressed. In man's primitive state, when life was being threatened, the body's reaction to stress was obviously beneficial, as it helped to keep the person alive when in danger. Even now, if we are in a life-threatening situation, the body's automatic reactions may save our lives. But today, much of the stress we feel is not due to life-threatening situations and is therefore inappropriate. The table below shows clearly how each of our body's responses can have a detrimental effect.

Physical Reactions of the Body under Stress

Natural response to stress	Benefits	Detrimental effects over prolonged periods of stress
Increase of thyroid hormone in the bloodstream	Speeds up the body's metabolism, providing extra energy to cope with the emergency at hand	Can lead to insomnia and exhaustion. May also cause an intolerance to heat and extreme nervousness.
Adrenal glands release cortisone	Protects the body from an allergic reaction such as asthma	Destroys the body's resistance to infection so that the ability to fight off illnesses is impaired. Makes bones more brittle so that they are more prone to fracture. Dramatically reduces the stomach's resistance to its own acid and can lead to gastric and duodenal ulcers.
Hypothalamus releases endorphins	Similar effects to morphine, killing pain so that the person under stress does not feel injuries until after the danger has passed	Depletes the levels of endorphins in the body and can aggravate painful conditions such as migraines, backaches, headaches and arthritis.
Release of sugar into the bloodstream, producing an increase in the insulin level	Provides a short-lived energy supply to enable the person to escape from a situation quickly	Excessive demands on the pancreas for insulin can bring about or aggravate diabetes.

Significant reduction in activity of the digestive system	Allows blood to be diverted from the digestive system to the muscles so that 'super-human' feats can be performed in times of danger	Eating 'fast foods' or grabbing a snack while under stress can do a lot of harm as the person forces foods into an inactive stomach. Can cause indigestion, nausea or cramps.
Increase of cholesterol in the blood	Gives the muscles energy over a prolonged period of stress	Over time, cholesterol deposits can cause hardening of the arteries, which may contribute to heart attacks.
Heartbeat rate increases	Pumps the blood faster to give the body more energy	May causes hypertension (high blood pressure) which could lead to strokes or heart attacks.
Rapid breathing	Supplies the blood with extra oxygen	The lungs take in a greater quantity of polluted air if you live in a city or if you smoke. Can also cause hyperventilation.
Thickening of the blood	Creates a greater capacity in the blood to carry oxygen, slows down bleeding from a wound and helps to fight infections	Increases the risk of heart attacks and strokes.
Increase in the activity of the sweat gland	Cools down the body which is hotter from over-exertion	Over-sweating/ increased body odour, clammy palms

Sight, hearing, touch, taste and smell all become more acute

When in danger it is vital that all the senses are functioning at their optimum to ensure survival

Senses are dulled after a stressful situation and errors in judgement can easily occur.

Stress and Fear

As we have seen, the physical effects of stress may start as early as five or six years of age, when children have to be at school on time or when they have to perform under test conditions. Children soon learn of the punishments and rewards they will receive if they fail or succeed, and the fear of failure at school, even at this early age, often brings about the habitual muscular tension and pulled-back head, hunched shoulders and shortened spine that most of us carry with us into adulthood. This in turn causes other muscles throughout the body to contract and tense, and produces the disturbing postures that are so common today.

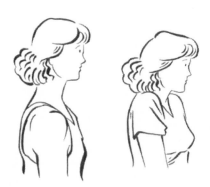

a) shoulders in normal, relaxed position;
b) shoulders hunched due to emotional stress

Faced with this fear of failure or of being late for school over a long period of time, the child's pattern of movement will become almost permanently over-tense, and this will in turn affect his or her behaviour. By the time the child reaches adulthood these habits will be firmly ingrained and will even feel completely normal and natural, in spite of the fact that they harm posture, produce aches and pains, restrict movement and even adversely affect the person's attitude to life.

As stress is clearly reflected in our posture and patterns of movement, the effects of stress can be reduced by changing the way we *use* ourselves. Even active adults who take part in yoga, sport or other physical training are not immune to detrimental postural habits and will, in fact, reinforce these harmful tendencies with every action they perform. Even if they realize that they do have poor posture, they will often try to improve it by doing what they were instructed to do at school, which was to 'sit up straight', by over-tightening the lower back muscles. The most common place for back problems is in the lower back, so it is not inconceivable that a large percentage of back problems can be attributed to the habit of over-tensing the lumbar area.

'Improving' Posture

The same kind of instructions continue to be given in our society today. We are told to sit or stand in a certain way in order to 'improve' our posture by people who, while trying to be helpful, are often suffering from faulty sensory perception themselves. Even if this is not the case and they are knowledgeable about how the body's reflexes work, and their students can understand what is being asked of them, there still remains the huge obstacle of faulty sensory perception on the part of the students themselves.

Very few people I have met - and this includes some physical education instructors, yoga teachers, ballet and other dance teachers, as well as some doctors, osteopaths, chiropractors and physiotherapists - are aware that their sensory perception, or kinaesthetic sense, is often unreliable. Without an awareness of this fact it is practically impossible to teach anyone how to improve the way they use themselves, whether it be their posture while standing or sitting, or the way they carry out more active movements such as walking, running, dancing or playing sport. In fact, when people try to improve their posture without knowledge about faulty sensory perception, they often make the situation worse instead of better by over-tightening muscles. I have come across several stress-relieving and posture-improving techniques which actually cause the muscular system to be under more strain than usual.

Modern Times

As recently as the 1950s, people had a more relaxed way of life and more quiet times, partly because the motor car, television, telephone and many other modern inventions had yet to make a significant impact on their lives.

> It is an interesting fact that in the US the average child of 10 has seen over 5,000 murders on television.

These days it is very rare for us to be alone with our own thoughts, and we are constantly encouraged to achieve more and more, until we have become a race of 'human doers' instead of 'human beings'. Many of us have even forgotten how just to *be*, and can get quite agitated when we have nothing to do.

We must learn to stop completely and become aware of the muscular tension we are holding even when we are supposedly doing nothing. Self-awareness is a basic tool to help you to relieve many of the ailments that life's stresses and strains have caused, and it is not until you become aware of your muscular tension that you can do anything about it. The following procedure is very simple, but can be extremely effective in reducing stress levels. It can also be helpful to those suffering from the muscular tension that causes backache, neck problems or headaches, which frequently accompany stress. In addition, it can help to align the spine and release the often undetected tension present in the neck and shoulders. If this procedure is to be effective it should be carried out on a daily basis.

Stress-reducing Method

When you first start using this, you may feel overwhelmed with thoughts of all the things you need to do, or even feelings of guilt; this can cause you to become restless or fidgety. This is quite normal, especially if you are under stress. Don't give up. After a week or so you may start to see the benefits. As your mind and body begin to calm down, you will actually become more efficient and will get more done in the long run.

Lie down on your back, place some thin *paperback* books under your head and put your hands gently on either side of your navel. Bring your feet up near your pelvis, so that your knees are bent and are pointing up to the ceiling. Your feet should be making even contact with the floor and there should be some space between them, as well as space between your knees. Direct your knees up towards the ceiling, so that they do not fall inwards or outwards.

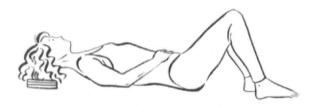

The main aim of this exercise is to release unwanted muscular tension throughout the body. It is far easier to let go of tension in this position because gravity is working on your body in a different way from when you are upright. The height of the books needed under the head will vary from person to person; the best way to find the exact number of books you need is to ask your Alexander teacher when you start having lessons.

Make sure that your head is not tilting backwards on to the books. As a general rule, it is better to have too many books than too few, but make sure your head is not pushed so far forward that it feels uncomfortable, or that your breathing is restricted. If you are still uncertain, it is probably best to use a pillow or cushion for the time being until you are able to see an Alexander teacher who can instruct you more accurately.

As Alexander discovered, most of us pull our heads back habitually and unconsciously, so having the books behind your head will begin to prevent this from happening. When first trying this semi-supine position, you may like to place a thin piece of foam or a towel on top of the books if that feels more comfortable. The reason you have your knees bent is so that you can more easily release tension in the lumbar region (lower back); in time you may find that your back gradually flattens on to the floor. Keep your eyes open throughout the procedure, as this will help you to remain in a state of alertness as you release unwanted tension.

Now, think of the following 'Directions' (*for more about Alexander's Directions, see Chapter 2*):

- *Think of your neck muscles lengthening and softening* so that any excess tension in your neck is released - this will help to free your head from your spine. You may also like to think of your head going forward and outward away from your spine, as this will help the spine to lengthen. Make sure you don't do it, just that you think of it.

- *Think of your back lengthening and widening on to the floor.* Again, it is very important that you do not do anything to make this happen, as this will simply tighten up the back muscles even more.

- *Think of your elbows releasing away from one another.* This will encourage freedom in the wrist and elbow joints, as well as helping to release tension in and around the shoulders. Make sure there is some space between your elbows and ribcage.

- *Imagine your shoulders widening away from one another.* This will release muscular tension in the upper part of the chest, which will improve your breathing. This Direction is particularly helpful to anyone with rounded shoulders.

- *Think of your right shoulder releasing away from your left hip and of your left shoulder releasing away from your right hip.* These two Directions can be very beneficial for releasing the shoulders backwards and for reducing tension around the ribcage and in the abdomen.

- *Think of your knees going up towards the ceiling.* This will help to release any tension you may be carrying in your legs. You may find it helpful to think of your knees being supported by imaginary strings which are attached to the ceiling.

- *Think of your toes lengthening as the soles of your feet spread out on to the floor.* This will help you to release tension in your toes and feet.

These are just a few of the Directions you can think about to help you release muscular tension. Improving the way you breathe (*see Chapter 8*) will also be of benefit.

It is important to remember that you must not do anything to find the right position: you merely send thought messages to the areas. The process of releasing tension depends on you *doing less*.

It may take a few weeks or more before you feel totally comfortable in the semi-supine position, so be patient. Initially it may be a good idea to practise this method for just 10 minutes each day. You can then increase by one minute a day until you have reached 20 minutes. If at any time you experience pain in your back or neck while going through this procedure, do not persevere. Simply get up and try again another time.

Benefits of the Semi-supine Position

Most people find that the following benefits arise only if this method is used on a regular basis (once a day for at least 15 minutes) over a period of some weeks. Try to do it halfway through your day; if this is not possible, do it whenever you can. You may find that you have an improved night's sleep if you do it just before going to bed, while other people feel that starting the day in this way suits them better, as they are aware of the benefits throughout the day. You may feel uncomfortable if you attempt the method after a heavy meal, and if this is the case it is best avoided. It is much harder to release tension if you are feeling cold or lying in a draught, so make sure you are warm enough and, if necessary, place a blanket over yourself.

When you are horizontal the spine is at rest; this is the best position in which to release any tension that may be present in the neck and back. When you are upright, the curves in the spine can sometimes be exaggerated which can shorten your stature; by lying down regularly you may find you have increased in height by an inch or two (2.5 - 5 cm). Lying down once a day helps to prevent unwanted tension from building up, thereby avoiding a whole range of problems later in life. Lying down in the semi-supine position may also help to slow down the process of wear and tear of the bones and joints.

Other benefits that can be gained by practising the semi-supine position are:

- a reduction in physical stress
- more energy to cope with daily life
- reduced muscular tension throughout the body
- a lengthened spine, allowing better support
- the release of tension from around the ribcage, improving breathing
- improved circulation (the blood can flow better through muscles that are relaxed)

- a more effective digestive system
- freeing of nerves that have become trapped due to over-tense muscles
- more room for the internal organs to function efficiently.

Although this process is very simple, many people tense their muscles even more when first starting to try to relax them. It is strongly advised that you see an Alexander Technique teacher to help you to notice which sensations accompany the reduction of muscle tension. When you are able to detect and release muscle tension while lying down, you may then practise the same *Directions* as you go about your daily activities. You may well find that other stressful symptoms disappear over a period of time as your bodily functions come back into balance.

A series of Alexander lessons is recommended in order for you to become used to the new ways of moving, otherwise there will be a tendency for you to revert back to your old habits.

Many people have said to me when they first do this exercise that it seems too simple to be really effective. They have usually been suffering for many years and have been to see doctors and specialists and tried a vast range of expensive operations or treatments, none of which has given any lasting relief. The Alexander Technique does not in itself claim to cure anything, but it does teach you how to stop interfering with your body's natural healing processes, and in this way the body may heal itself.

4
Worry

What lies behind us, and what lies before us are tiny matters compared to what lies within us.

Ralph Waldo Emerson

There is no such thing as a 'born worrier'. No one spends their first moments of life fearing the future or regretting the past. Worrying is simply a mental habit that the mind acquires, and with determination and faith in ourselves we can eradicate it from our lives.

The tendency to worry develops with age, and can affect us physically and emotionally as well as mentally. If it goes unchecked, worry can eventually go on to cause serious damage to our health - then we really will have something to worry about!

If the habit of worrying is allowed to take hold, we can become constantly haunted by all the possible scenarios of what might or might not happen. Worry can affect our sleeping patterns and deprive us of the necessary recharging mechanisms that our body needs for good health. It is important to realize that, as with any other habit, this one can be broken; the only requirements are patience and a resolve to stop worrying and start enjoying this precious life. If you are able to gain control over your worries about achieving goals you will cultivate patience, which in turn will create confidence, decisiveness and a calm, rational outlook on life.

Financial Worry

Today, financial worry seems to be far more common than ever before, even though many of us have far greater financial security than our ancestors or people in other cultures.

A great many of us are convinced that all our problems would be solved if we could only win the lottery or come by a great deal of money from some other source. It may be a cliché, but riches can bring additional worries: that we will be burgled, for example, or that those we trust with handling our wealth will abuse their position for personal gain. Unless we have the time and space to examine the root cause of our own personal habit of worrying, no amount of money or possessions will alter it.

Hint

Is it not strange that just when you solve one problem, another one immediately takes its place?

The Origin of Worry

Worrying is a habit that, once ingrained, forces our mind into overdrive even when there is nothing to worry about. As our mind becomes overactive it will imagine a whole range of disastrous possibilities, even though we know from past experience that the probability of many of these ever happening is very remote. In a great variety of ways society encourages us to think and prepare for the future, and these concerns are exacerbated by the advertisements for personal pensions, income protection plans and a wide range of 'future planning' policies. We are actively encouraged to worry - in the mistaken belief that we will thus be prepared for any disaster that befalls us. But no matter how much worrying we do, it does not help one iota when disaster does come; in fact, quite the reverse - a person with a happy and positive outlook on life is far more likely to cope with a crisis than one who is pessimistic.

Tip

To beat the worrying habit we need to understand on a very deep level that unless we attend to each and every moment we are missing the rich and wonderful experience of living.

It is now commonplace for people to fret if they don't know exactly what is going to happen during each moment of their day. This leaves very little room for spontaneity, which is a necessary ingredient in a healthy, happy life. As a result, many people are not excited with life and blame their boredom on their job, their relationships, or the place where they live. Yet we did not start life this way. As children, we all knew instinctively how to live in the present moment and get the most out of everything we did, and as a result we were much happier. Watch a young child playing with the simplest toy - a stick or a cardboard box, say. She will play excitedly for hours, unaware even that time exists. If you ask young children about what they are going to do tomorrow, most will have no idea, unless this has been impressed upon them by their parents or society. If we have a tendency to plan ahead constantly, we will be more likely to worry when things do not fit into our scheme of things. John Lennon summed it up very well when he said that life is what happens to you while you're busy making other plans. The message is clear: enjoy each day as it comes.

Choose a day when you do not have to go to work and you have no prior commitments, possibly during a holiday or at the weekend. Do not plan anything for that day. Wake up and just take the day as it comes. Only do things you enjoy, rather that activities or chores that you should or must do. If you please yourself for the whole day, you will probably find that your mind will make several attempts to make you feel guilty - if you can, observe those thoughts and feelings objectively without being taken in by them. You may like to write down any thoughts and feelings that emerge throughout the day. Some people find this simple exercise very difficult at first, because they are so conditioned to planning every aspect of their lives that they feel most uncomfortable when they do not have a goal. They even begin to worry about not finding anything with which to occupy their day. After trying this simple exercise a few times, you will realize that you can enjoy life far more with the minimum of planning.

Worry and Illness

Many of our worries concern other people, but you'd do everyone a favour by being less concerned about the past or future. In the same way that happiness is infectious, so is worry. By worrying less you will not only feel more contented, but you will also make your home and workplace happier environments for both yourself and others. When I am teaching people about how the Alexander Technique can help them to let go of their worries and truly enjoy themselves, many of them begin to feel that they are being selfish or self-centred. They have been taught from an early age that it is wrong to spend time not being concerned about others. In reality, if we are over-controlled by worry we may well become ill as a result, and will then actually be a burden on our family, friends and co-workers.

It is estimated that as many as 30 per cent of people in the US have suffered at some point from a nervous breakdown caused by worry (as cited in Dale Carnegie's *How to Stop Worrying and Start Living*). Worry can also cause muscle tension which, as we have already seen, can result in backache, migraines, hypertension and a wide range of physical disorders. Dr Alexis Carrel, winner of the Nobel prize for medicine, said 'Businessmen who do not know how to fight worry die young' - in other words, worry can not only ruin life as we live it, but will shorten it as well. He went on to say that those people who can maintain inner peace in the midst of turmoil are immune from nervous disorders.

Longevity

The more you worry, the greater the chance of your being inflicted with an illness that will shorten your life. There are a great many cases demonstrating that over-worry can cause or exacerbate ulcers, heart disease, strokes or even fatal accidents through lack of concentration. One of the oldest people on record was a Japanese man by the name of Shigechiyo Izumi. He lived to be over 119 years of age and was convinced that the reason for his longevity was that he refused to let anything worry him.

If you knew that this was your last day on earth, how much would you give for another month? Another week? Or even just one more day? You would probably give everything you own just for an extra hour, especially as we all know that we cannot take anything with us when we go. But how often do we really appreciate this life compared to how much time we spend struggling to become better off, to succeed, to achieve something that so often is unsatisfying and unrewarding when we actually get it? Look back at your life and ask yourself what were the highlights: Was it really driving the new car for the first time so that you could show it off to your neighbours? The delivery of the three-piece suite you had saved up for so long to buy? Or working at that well-paid job? Most of these experiences fade within a few weeks, while the lasting memories are of gestures of love and kindness that people have shown us and that we have shown others. Maybe at the end of our days we will finally realize that these are the things that really matter ... but by then it will too late.

If we remain continually worried about something or other we are in effect missing out on our true potential, because we are not actually present to experience our life as it passes - we are merely entertaining one silly thought after another. At the end of life we do not want to be left with regrets, as underscored in this poem by Nadine Stair:

> *If I had my life to live over, I'd try to make more mistakes next time.*
> *I would relax. I would limber up.*
> *I would be sillier than I have been on this trip.*
> *I know of very few things I would take seriously. I would be crazier.*
> *I would be less hygienic. I would take more chances.*
> *I would take more trips. I would climb more mountains, swim*
> *more rivers and watch more sunsets.*
> *I would eat more ice cream and less beans.*
> *I would have more actual troubles and fewer imaginary ones.*
> *You see, I am one of those people who lives prophylactically and*
> *sanely and sensibly, hour after hour, day after day.*
> *Oh, I have had my moments and, if I had to do it over again,*

I'd have more of them. In fact, I'd try to have nothing else.
Just moments, one after another, instead of living so many years
ahead each day.
I have been one of those people who never go anywhere without a
thermometer, a hot water bottle, a gargle, a raincoat and a para-
chute.
If I had it to do over again, I would go places and do things and
travel lighter than I have.
If I had my life to live over, I would start barefoot earlier in the
spring and stay that way later in the fall. I would play hooky more.
I wouldn't make such good grades except by accident.
I would ride on more merry-go-rounds.
I'd pick more daisies.

But there is a way that we can change the way we live today. All we really need to do is put everything into its true perspective rather than seeing it as most other people do. Deep in our hearts we know what we have to do to achieve a long and fulfilling life - the problem is that we have forgotten how fortunate we really are.

Tip

Just stand back for a moment and ask yourself 'How precious am I really?'

The Power of the Mind

The mind is much more powerful than many of us realize. More that 300 years ago, the great poet Milton wrote these lines:

The mind is its own place, and in itself Can make a heaven of Hell,
a hell out of Heaven

The following true accounts are living proof of how powerful our thoughts can be.

Jennifer was diagnosed with cancer after going to her doctor for some routine tests. Understandably she became very distraught, which obviously did not help her condition, and she deteriorated rapidly. Very soon she was bedridden, as she became weaker and weaker and eventually suffered all the awful symptoms of cancer. Over a period of several months she was unable to eat very much, lost over 25 kg in weight and was eventually moved into a hospice for the dying. She was a shadow of her former self and everyone, including herself, expected her to die any day. Just at this point, the hospital contacted the hospice to inform her that they had mixed up the records: she did not have cancer after all. She immediately started to regain weight and her health quickly returned. She then set about suing her local health authority for destroying her life.

In direct contrast, the second account concerns Jim, a widower who was diagnosed as being in the advanced stages of cancer. His doctor estimated that Jim had only a month to live. Jim left the doctor's surgery in shock and walked over to a nearby park. He thought for a long time about his life. On his way home he stopped at the travel agent's and enquired about cruises round the Caribbean. The only one available was a six-week excursion due to set sail in a week's time. Nevertheless, Jim booked himself a berth. He had a most wonderful time on his cruise and returned six weeks later feeling better than he had for many years. He went for further tests and completely baffled his doctor because there was now not a sign of cancer in his body. Overjoyed, he left the surgery and went on to live a rich and full life. If he had let worry eat away at him rather than make a last effort to enjoy himself, things might have turned out differently.

These two examples show clearly how powerful the mind can be. In some circumstances it can literally kill us; in others, it can allow us to lead a wonderful, happy life. It all depends on how much control we have over it. If we are pessimistic, it follows that life will be hard and sad; we will see everything as an effort and will eventually wear ourselves out. If, on the other hand, we are optimistic, life will be so much easier and will present many more exciting possibilities. It's all a question of perspective. Of course, the way we perceive the world depends on our prior conditioning and past experiences, but at any moment in time we can, with consciousness and common sense, change the way we see the world. All we have to do is decide to throw away the habits of a lifetime. This is easier than it seems, and is certainly worth it when you stop to consider what's at stake - the quality of your life.

Exercise

The following exercise demonstrates the power that our mind has over us and the interconnection between the body, mind and emotions.

You might want to tape-record the passages that follow, or you and a friend can take it in turns reading them aloud to one another.

Find a place where you can lie down and relax without any interruptions. Now close your eyes and listen:

Imagine it is your first day at a new job. It is a job you have wanted for a long time and you want to get to your place of work early to make a good impression. You know the traffic is bad on a Monday morning, so you plan to leave the house in plenty of time and decide you will drive to the station and catch the train. Imagine you wake up that morning and for some reason your alarm clock has failed to go off. You have overslept by half an hour and now have just enough time for a quick wash and a hasty breakfast. While you are in the bathroom the phone rings and, although at first you think you'll just let it ring, it goes on for so long that eventually you pick up, thinking it might be something urgent. It is a good friend who is very distressed and you are caught on the phone for 10 minutes or more. You are looking constantly at your watch and realize that you must leave within the next few minutes if you are to catch your train. You eventually get off the phone and dash out to the car, only to realize that you've left the lights on all night and the battery is flat. You rush down to the end of the road hoping to catch a taxi, and as luck would have it you manage to find one. When you get out at the station, however, to your horror you realize that in your haste you have left your money on the table at home. The taxi driver can't accept credit cards but is very understanding, and asks you to write down your name and address so that he can call round later for the fare. You finally dash on to the platform - only to see your train pulling out of the station!

Now keep still and do not open your eyes. Feel if there is any reaction within your body. Can you detect any tension in your muscles? Are you feeling any different emotionally? How are you breathing? You may like to write down your observations. After about five minutes lie down and close your eyes again and listen to this second passage:

Imagine you are lying on the beach in Hawaii. It has been a hot day, but now it is evening and the temperature is perfect. You can feel the warm sand underneath you and hear the sound of the waves as they lap on the shore. There is also a warm breeze and you become aware of the sound it is making in the trees nearby. In the far distance you can hear the sound of children's laughter. You decide to go into the water and you walk down the gently slopping shore until the water laps around your feet and ankles. You sit down and feel the sensation of the warm, clear water all around you. A friend comes up to you and offers to go and fetch you a long, cool fruit juice while you stay and watch the bright orange sun sink slowly towards the horizon. You have an overwhelming feeling that life is good and wish you could stay in this place of tranquillity for ever.

Again, do not move; simply focus on what you are feeling. When you are ready, write it all down. In reality, you have not left the room except in your thoughts, but you've probably noticed that the two passages produced very different reactions in your body.

This exercise demonstrates that the mind, body and emotions cannot be separated and that your thoughts alone can produce feelings of stress or, alternatively, relaxation.

The Precious Present

It is important to realize that there is a difference between discomfort and discontentment. If you are discontented with your life it does not matter what material comforts you have, you will still have a feeling that something is wrong. If you lie awake at night feeling worried and stressed it really makes little difference how many pillows you have, how soft or hard the bed is or how warm or cold you are. Discomfort can be alleviated by material things, but discontentment cannot.

The only way we can become truly happy is to stop being concerned about the future or the past and start focusing on the only thing that is really happening - the here and now. Nobody knows what the future holds and no one can change the past, but we can do so much with each day as it comes. In fact, the way we live each day may heal the wounds of past experiences and set the foundations for the future. We will never get back even one second, so we need to take care of today. Most people have heard the words of Omar Khayyam:

> *The Moving Finger writes; and having writ,*
> *Moves on: nor all of your Piety or Wit*
> *Shall lure it back to cancel half a line,*
> *Nor all your Tears wash out a Word of it.*

You are alive and something is keeping you alive every second of your life - something is causing your breath to go in and out, but you never worry about that because something is taking care of it. The very same thing that is keeping you alive will also look after every other aspect of your life - if you let it.

Tip

Do yourself a favour - forget about yesterday and let tomorrow take care of itself.

Breaking the Habit of Worry

At this point you may well be thinking that it is all very well to talk about not worrying and living in the present, but that it is easier said than done. This is where the Alexander Technique comes into its own, because it helps in a practical way to quieten down an overactive mind. It is an unique tool for enabling us to be much more conscious, not only of how we use our bodies, but also how we use our minds and the way in which we react to our environment.

Alexander often referred to 'the mind wandering habit' that many people are afflicted with. He taught many of his pupils to use their thoughts constructively rather than destructively, by encouraging them to be aware of themselves and their immediate surroundings. When we are able to concentrate on being attentive as we perform each action, it is possible to channel our thoughts away from the future or past and into the 'here and now'. In the process of becoming a more conscious human being, you will start to notice how often your mind is in complete control of you, instead of the other way round. If you had an arm or leg that you were unable to control, you would not hesitate to seek medical help, yet the mind can be totally out of control and we may carry on for years hardly noticing this - or realizing that we can do something about it - at all.

It has been said that the mind is an incredible gift from our creator, but what we choose to think about is our gift to ourselves. If we worry constantly it is a sign that the mind is dominating our lives and that there is an urgent need to bring it back under control in order to use it as the incredible tool it was designed to be. We can only think one conscious thought at a time, so if we train our mind to attend to how we think and behave from moment to moment, our worried thoughts will soon diminish. The mind can easily slip into the past or future, but the body can only exist in this very instant; by focusing on how we use the physical body we can become more focused on the present moment. As a result, we will be able to exercise more control over our mind and ultimately ourselves. This process will lead us to become more fulfilled and have a more enjoyable life.

Tip

When we are able to accept life just the way it is rather than wishing it were different, then true happiness is attainable.

Practical Steps to Prevent Worry

It is not easy fro people who are prone to worry to stop their minds wandering, because they have become so used to listening to the negative thoughts that continually bombard their mind. From an early age many of us have paid attention to the external stimuli which continually attract our mind away from the present moment. Paying attention to the way we are performing our everyday actions will help to bring us back to the 'here and now' rather than let our minds take us to the past or future. A practical way we can attend to our actions is to use Inhibition and Alexander's Directions.

Worry and Inhibition

As we saw in Chapter 2, Alexander discovered that without *Inhibition* it was impossible for him to change any of his habits even once he had recognized them. Through this process of stopping and consciously choosing a different way of reacting, we can gain greater control over the mind-wandering thoughts which can plague us throughout our lives. For people who use the Alexander Technique, Inhibition has a very definite purpose: it helps to prevent unconsidered and conditioned responses, probably learned in childhood, which are now no longer appropriate. A moment's pause gives us an opportunity to prevent our mind from worrying and instead to begin a reasoned consideration of the situation. This will heighten our awareness, making conscious choice possible and providing us with a chance to react in a more positive, healthy way.

In stressful situations our 'fear reflexes' are triggered, causing us to pull the head back and down on to the spine and hunch the shoulders - this is sometimes known as the 'startle pattern'. If we are constantly worried, our entire muscular system and co-ordination of movement are continually being interfered with. This muscular tension can prevent us from thinking clearly. Inhibition can help us to remain poised and calm even when something serious is troubling us.

Tip

Knowing how to wait is often thought to be the secret of success.

Inhibition is the key to changing all kinds of habits and can also be essential when combating worry, because it can give you time to consider the following points which can help you to get to the root of your worries:

- What are you actually worried about?
- What are the chances of the thing you are worried about actually happening?
- What is the worst thing that could actually happen to you?
- What can you do practically to prevent what you fear from actually happening?

What Am I Actually Worried About?

This is often not as obvious as it may at first seem. Take, for instance, the fear of unemployment. Even if a person dislikes their work, they can suffer from this worry. The underlying fear could be loss of status or independence, of being pitied by one's family, friends or neighbours. Pride may come into it, as well as the bald fact of not having money coming in regularly, or having to adjust to a much lower wage. Pinpointing the underlying fear is the first step to overcoming it.

What Are the Chances of the Thing You Are Worried about Actually Happening?

Take a look at all the things you have been worried about in the past and ask yourself how many of them have actually happened. Most of our worries will never manifest and in retrospect are simply a waste of time and energy. How many times have you thought afterwards that you were worrying over nothing?

What Is the Worst Thing that Could Actually Happen to You?

Whatever horrors your imagination can throw up, especially in the small hours when the smallest problem seems insurmountable, spending any amount of time worrying about them achieves nothing (apart, perhaps, from making you ill). Worrying beforehand about a 'worst-case scenario' won't change a thing. Think of times when you have correctly anticipated something dreadful happening, compared with times when you haven't - did you feel any better in either case? Were your reactions different? Instead of dwelling on what might happen, far better to put your energy towards living in the moment.

What Can You Do Practically to Prevent What You Fear from Actually Happening?

If there is a practical situation that is causing you distress, try to work out if there is any way you can improve it. Often, if we are calm we can think of a solution. Talking over your concerns with a friend or counsellor can sometimes be a great help.

If you can do nothing about the situation, just accept it. You'll find that changing your attitude towards it will make a real difference. Remember, too, that rushing into situations without thinking about the consequences frequently causes further problems which could otherwise have been avoided.

Tip

It is sometimes useful to try to recall what we were worried about a year ago - more often than not we cannot remember unless we ask friends or family, or perhaps if we've kept a diary or some other record. Worries soon pass, to be replaced by new ones - unless we choose another path.

Unless we can learn how to pause before acting and bring our thoughts away from past and future matters, we will never be able stop worrying and start enjoying life, and we may even be afflicted with stress-related health problems. Many people find Inhibition the most difficult aspect of the Alexander Technique to put into practice. They feel that they hardly have time to think while they are under pressure to complete a number of activities in a limited time. The concept of pausing before we act seems almost incomprehensible, yet as the pace of life increases this ability to pause becomes ever more important. If you do not think clearly when you make your decisions they will more often than not be inappropriate ones.

Is it not strange that there is hardly ever enough time to do a job properly, but we can always find time to go back afterwards and correct the mistakes?

Worry and Directions

By thinking of the Directions (as explained in *Chapter 2, 'Changing the Pattern of Thought'*), you will not only be able to release muscular tension and perform everyday actions more efficiently, but will also have a place to focus your mind on something that is happening in the present moment. As you practise thinking of your body releasing tension, your mind will be engaged in a practical way and be unable to fill you with fear about the future. The more you practise the art of bringing your mind back to your immediate surroundings, and to how you are performing everyday actions, the easier it will be to break the habit of worrying.

Make sure, however, that you do not start to worry about whether you are thinking about the *correct* Directions in the right way! Your Alexander teacher will be able to tell you which Directions are most beneficial for you individually, but it is always necessary to think of freeing your neck, so that your head can go forward and up and therefore your whole spine can lengthen. After continual practice of these and other Directions, you will be in more control of your wandering mind rather than it being in control of you.

Freedom of Choice

Alexander was adamant that the goal of his Technique was to give each and every human being the power to choose. He believed that unless people are able to think for themselves and make decisions based on what they want in life, rather that what everyone else wants from them, they can never really be fulfilled.

When we look around us, we see people trying to be the same as others around them rather than making their own informed choices. Without Alexander's form of Inhibition there can be no change - our mind-wandering habits will prevail, and if we do what we have always done we will obviously get the same results as we have always got in the past. It's up to you. Only you can take up the opportunities being offered - no one can do that for you. If you have a strongly ingrained habit of worrying, just reading this book may not be enough, and you will need the help of a qualified Alexander Technique teacher who will show you how to release tension and practise Inhibition in a practical way. In the mean time, however, you might like to try putting the good advice of Sibyl Partridge into practice:

Just for today I will be happy.
Most people are about as happy as they make up their minds to be.
Happiness is from within, it is not a matter of externals.
Just for today I will try to adjust myself to what is, and not try
to adjust everything to my own desires. I will take my family, my
business, and my luck as they come and fit myself to them.
Just for today, I will take good care of my body. I will exercise it,
care for it, nourish it, not abuse it, nor neglect it, so that it will be a
perfect machine for my bidding.
Just for today, I will try to strengthen my mind, I will learn some-
thing useful. I will not be a mental loafer. I will read something
that requires effort, thought and concentration.
Just for today I will do someone a good turn and not get found out.
Just for today I will be agreeable. I will look as well as I can, dress

*as becomingly as possible, talk low, act courteously, be liberal with
praise, criticize not at all, not find fault with anything and not try
to regulate nor improve anyone.*

*Just for today I will try to live this day only, and not try to tackle
my whole life problems at once.*

*Just for today I will have a programme, I will write down what I
hope to do every hour. I may not follow it exactly, but I will have it.
It will eliminate two pests, hurry and indecision.*

*Just for today I will have a quiet half-hour all by myself and relax.
In this half an hour I will think of God, so as to get a little more
perspective into my life.*

*Just for today I will be unafraid, especially I will not be afraid to be
happy, to enjoy what is beautiful, to love, and to believe that those I
love, love me.*

Tip

Remember: Your mind is a gift from the creator, but what you think
about is your gift to yourself. Don't you think that you deserve better?

5
Anxiety

Life is not an emergency

Ram Dass

Anxiety can be seen as a stage further on from worry. An overactive mind brings on the state of extreme tension present in such a condition. Those who suffer from extreme anxiety have usually had an abundance of goals and deadlines in their lives and can no longer cope. They have become used to living under great strain, to the extent that their minds and bodies are habitually stressed. This kind of mental tension can lead to panic attacks - clear warning signs that steps need to be taken before matters get any worse. Often, however, those suffering from panic attacks can feel so overwhelmed that they do not know where to begin finding help.

When something in our lives is not working we normally take the time to find out why; for example, each time we turn the key in the ignition to start the car we automatically wait to hear the engine before we put it into gear. If for some reason the engine does not start, we naturally try to find out why or seek help. We apply this simple logic to everything we do in our lives, but somehow we do not apply the same common sense when our very life is not working out in the way we want it to. When suffering from acute anxiety, many people become so involved in trying to get their life under control that they find it difficult to stop and think in order to find the root cause of the problem. If you suffer from anxiety or panic attacks, it is imperative that you examine your life in order to find an easier and more simple way of living. 'Impossible, you do not understand my situation,' I hear you say; well, your body is telling you in no uncertain terms to stop and take stock or your life, and probably make some big changes. There is a solution to your problem; there is a way of creating an easier, more enjoyable life for yourself, but if you are ever going to find the answer you must first realize just how important you are.

What Is a Panic Attack?

Fear is a normal reaction to danger. As we have seen in previous chapters, anxiety takes place when your life is being threatened in some way. In fact, if you were confronted by a ferocious dog and you *didn't* experience fear, there would be something wrong with you. People who suffer from panic attacks have similar responses - only in their case there is often no apparent reason for them to become afraid. They may be simply walking along the street or queuing in a post office with no immediate danger present and suddenly a panic attack happens without warning. The reason for the onset of these attacks is that the anxiety in their mind becomes so acute that their body starts to display all the physical symptoms of stress. These people often struggle on, hoping that one day their fortunes will change and somehow or other the attacks will cease as suddenly as they started. This is rarely the case. Everybody aims to be happy in life, yet people who suffer from such attacks live continually in a prison of anxiety and fear.

When a panic attack first occurs it can be a very alarming experience, because the person can be totally unaware of what is happening. After this first attack the person concerned can then become frightened of having others in the future, and this fear itself can often bring on another attack. After each crisis the person will become more and more afraid of going back into situations which remind them of previous attacks. In other words, they actually become afraid of fear itself. The condition is self-perpetuating. They find themselves in fear of having an attack in public in case they make a fool of themselves. If these attacks are not dealt with, the sufferers will then start to lose confidence in themselves and may become reclusive.

During a panic attack you may experience one or more of the following physical symptoms:

- rapid heart rate or palpitations

- discomfort or pain in the chest

- shortness of breath

- sweating

- faintness or dizziness

- lack of co-ordination or feeling unsteady

- trembling or shakiness

- nausea

- numbness or tingling in the fingers or toes

- feeling of unreality

The mental and emotional states that accompany these sensations are:

- fear of losing control

- fear of death

- fear of madness

- a sudden and overwhelming feeling of terror or apprehension

- a sense of impending doom

Some sufferers may display only one or two of these symptoms, while others who are acutely affected can have a whole range.

In my experience, people are rarely suffering from panic attacks for the reason they think. They believe that their fear is caused by having to deal with certain situations, and although this is partly true, the real reason for the initial onset of panic attacks is a culmination of stress, tension and anxiety over many months, or perhaps even years. In other words, their body has become so used to living under stress that they no longer notice its effects; then, during the stressful period leading up to the attacks, the body and mind become extremely agitated, until eventually the person starts to experience detrimental behavioural reactions. These can include over-tensing of the entire muscular system, mental agitation, extreme mood swings, or emotional absence. These reactions start to occur for no reason and soon become part of the person's personality. Like worry, these habits become more ingrained as time goes on and, although some people may function in this state for many years, eventually the neuro-muscular system is under so much pressure that it can no longer cope with the strain. As a result, the systems throughout the body become more and more stressed until one day an attack of fear starts - seemingly 'out of nowhere'.

Panic Attacks and the Primary Control

In stressful situations or panic attacks, the muscle tension caused by the 'fight or flight' reflex causes interference with what Alexander called the Primary Control (*see Chapter 2*).

Specific physiological changes that take place during the fight or flight response include:

- the adrenal glands become more active
- the heart rate increases
- the breathing becomes more rapid
- the entire muscular system becomes tense
- the pupils dilate
- the level of sugar in the blood increases.

These changes make us more alert and ready to cope with the emergency at hand; when the danger has passed our body's functions gradually return to normal. Take note that these physiological changes are identical to the sensations experienced by panic attack sufferers.

If we are under constant stress at work, school or at home, the Primary Control is continually being interfered with and eventually this tension in the neck muscles becomes habitual, even when we are not under pressure. This interference is transmitted to other muscles throughout the body, producing a lack of balance and co-ordination and often resulting in excessive muscular tension, perhaps even causing the body to wear out before its time. By having Alexander Technique lessons you can learn how to release muscular tension and thus allow the Primary Control to work as nature intended; this in turn can help you to achieve a calmer and more relaxed outlook on life.

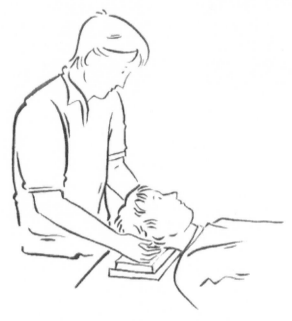

Freeing the neck which allows the Primary Control to work as it should

Secret Fears

The actual number of people who suffer from panic attacks is hard to calculate, as many of them keep their predicament a secret even from close friends and family. This is because they feel too ashamed to share their problem, as they are *afraid* of the embarrassment, ridicule or alienation that being open and honest might cause. This only adds to their feelings of isolation. A conservative estimate suggests that well over half a million people suffer regularly from these attacks in the UK alone, and this number is rising. According to Christine Ingham's book Panic Attacks, it is likely that over 20 million people in the UK, nearly 9 million in Australia and a staggering 87 million people in the US have experienced panic attacks. Most of these people have their first attack in adolescence or in their early twenties, although attacks have been known in children as young as four years old. The social pressures of having to achieve, acquire or perform at school, college or at work, as well as an increasingly unsettled home life may be the triggers which set off attack. Most adolescents who suffer panic attacks will, however, be likely to keep their experiences to themselves, for fear of admitting that there is 'something wrong' with them.

As with any other habit, the longer attacks have been occurring, the harder the cycle is to break. The fear of these attacks can affect the sufferer's quality of life to such an extent that some feel that life is simply not worth living.

Anxiety - and certainly a panic attack - is a clear indication that the person affected has been overdoing it and as a result their entire body and mind are constantly on 'red alert'. Their body is saying that rest is needed, and if they carry on without radically changing the way they live that rest may be forced upon them by nature in the form of a nervous or mental breakdown. Unfortunately, to add to the problem their body and mind are in such a state of anxiety that they are unable to 'switch off', so it is often impossible for them to get the vital rest they need. In other words, the person no longer possesses the natural ability to relax. Whenever they are in a state of panic it is extremely difficult for them to use their mind as a positive tool to extricate themselves from the predicament they are in. They feel that they are helpless victims and often rely on others to help them escape from the anguish they are experiencing. Although they need as much support as they can get through these troubled times, it is imperative that they realize that no one else can help them take responsibility for their condition. They need to be determined to deal with the problem; by so doing they can return to a normal way of life.

Body - Mind Unity

Most of the stress we feel today which leads to extreme anxiety originates in our minds; our thoughts are powerful enough to produce a physical or emotional reaction which we feel we can do little about. Alexander was convinced that the body, mind and emotions should be treated as a whole and not looked upon as separate entities. Even Hippocrates stated thousands of years ago that the treatment of physical symptoms without consideration of the patient's mental and emotional state would be completely ineffective. Yet today, when there is so much more medical knowledge, it is often only the physical symptoms that are given consideration.

In order to tackle the vicious circle of anxiety or panic we have become trapped in, we first need to look at the way we think. As we saw in Chapter 1, most young children experience only minimal tension, as can be seen by watching the freedom with which they move and use their bodies. It is only when their freedom to choose is removed that they too will start to feel the effects of stress, which is then reflected in their movements and posture. It is fear which reduces our freedom of choice. Some common childhood fears include:

- being late for school
- failing tests or examinations
- not progressing to higher levels of education

- not being able to find a job at the end of their education
- being ridiculed
- not being popular
- not being good enough.

If we compare these fears with those we experience as adults, you will see that there are some striking similarities:

- being late for work
- not meeting the targets at work
- unemployment
- not having enough money when we retire
- not being able to pay the bills
- not being accepted
- fear of inadequacy.

Fear of Failure

These fears can only be overcome if we begin to reverse the process which has led us to feel that we must avoid failure at all costs. Failure is part of the learning process of life, and in fact more can often be learned from failure than from success. It is also extremely important to separate the failure in our actions from any sense of personal failure. The fear of failure can often cause us to be so tense that failure becomes the inevitable consequence of our actions. This can be seen clearly when people are sitting exams, performing on stage or during job interviews. In fact, I used to witness the effects of fear of failure when I taught people to drive, as I regularly saw many capable young drivers fail their driving test simply because they became so anxious about being judged on their performance that they made silly mistakes. I even saw one or two of my pupils 'freeze with fear', unable even to start the car.

Before children go to school they may get frustrated when they are unable to do a certain activity, but they do not take it personally. They do not associate their inability to perform that task with the same deep-rooted feeling of failure that adults experience. When adults fail they can often feel that their whole life is a failure, and it is becoming more common for people to become very depressed or even commit suicide if, for example, they lose their job or their relationship ends.

Responsibility

It is true that we have more responsibility as we grow older. This, we may say, accounts for the feeling of a burden on our shoulders, and if we pause for a moment to think about the long list of things we are responsible for it is no wonder that we often feel stressed:

- mortgage or rent
- maintenance of flat or house
- home insurance
- government taxes
- car tax and insurance
- utility bills (gas, water, electricity)
- food and clothing for ourselves and our family
- work commitments
- family commitments

There is one responsibility missing from the list, however: responsibility to ourselves. We are responsible for our own happiness, though imposed guilt feelings often stop us from putting ourselves first. The reality is that if we did not exist all the other things to which we give so much importance would either not exist at all, or be perfectly well looked after by someone else. As already mentioned, many of us have been conditioned to think that it is selfish, and therefore wrong, to do things that make us happy. This is really not the case, because if we are content then everyone around us will benefit from the good feelings that we are experiencing. One of the main reasons people give for not having Alexander lessons is that they cannot justify spending the money on something that solely benefits themselves, but in reality if you look after yourself you will be better equipped to take care of others as well. I have often been told by my pupils that their having lessons has been instrumental in creating a more harmonious household. By directing our efforts solely to provide for our family's physical requirements, we often fail to provide them with what they need most.

When a person suffers from panic attacks it is not their physical health alone that needs to be dealt with, but their mental and emotional state as well. It is just as important to deal with issues of poor self-esteem or an overactive mind as it is to help release muscular tension. Although tranquillizers or sleeping pills may temporarily alleviate some of the physical symptoms of panic attacks, they will not help to get to the root of the problem.

Exercise

If you suffer from acute anxiety, you may like to try the following experiment to see if it is caused by a feeling that you have little choice in your life. Over a two-week period, choose a time every day that suits and spend a minimum of 30 minutes doing something you really enjoy. It may be a leisurely bath, a walk in the park or reading a book - you may like to do the same activity each day or you may choose to vary the things you do. It is important that you do not miss a day. After two weeks see, if you feel less stressed and more relaxed than you did previously. Nearly everyone has to do things that they dislike, but we need to balance these with things we enjoy. Most people I know who have tried this exercise have found that the more they do in their life that they truly enjoy, the less stressed they become.

Being Honest with Yourself

If you suffer from panic attacks, it is of primary importance that you face up to the problem openly. As you can see from the statistics mentioned above, you are not alone with your problem and there is help available to you. Keeping your attacks a secret will only either make them more intense or prolong their duration.

What happens to you during a panic attack is a natural reaction to danger - a normal response to a situation which makes you afraid. The panic you experience is your body's pre-programmed way of reacting to that danger. When this reaction is activated normally it could actually save your life, so in reality you have nothing to fear from these attacks as they are primarily a survival mechanism.

What is *not* normal, however, is the fact that these fear reflexes become activated for no apparent reason. The actual reason for the initial occurrence is that you have probably been in a state of fear and anxiety for a lengthy period of time *prior* to the attacks, and have formed a habit of tensing your muscles, even when there is nothing to be anxious about.

First and most importantly, you need to realize that although panic attacks are extremely unpleasant and frightening there is no evidence that any harm has come to anyone because of them, and therefore contrary to what you are experiencing during one of these attacks, your safety is *not* being threatened.

Secondly, it is important to tell your family or close friends about the attacks you are having, so that they can understand what is happening to you and give you their support. If the attacks are especially traumatic, it is also advisable to see your doctor so that he or she can prescribe helpful medication in the short term. This will help you to alleviate the symptoms until such a time when you feel able to deal with the fundamental cause of your attacks using the Alexander Technique.

Thirdly, when you suffer from a panic attack it is important to realize that the experience you are having will soon pass and that the attacks themselves will become less frequent with time until they will disappear altogether. The less you are frightened of them, the quicker this will happen.

Lastly, it may be helpful for you to think on the enlightened words of Richard Bach (in his book Illusions): "'There is no such thing as a problem without a gift for you in its hands.'" - This is your opportunity to find that gift!

How the Alexander Technique Can Help

The Alexander Technique does not offer a 'quick fix' solution for alleviating the symptoms of panic attacks. What is needed is a re-education of the muscular and nervous system, and this will take time. The best way forward to achieving lasting results is to have lessons from a qualified Alexander teacher (see 'Useful Addresses' at the end of this book).

'Letting Go'

You can help yourself immediately, however, by doing the semi-supine procedure as described in Chapter 2. If done regularly on a daily basis it may help you to release muscular tension and gradually prevent the over-stimulation of the nervous system. The most useful Directions that are particularly useful are the ones that directly affect the Primary Control:

- Allow there to be freedom of your neck.
- Allow your head to go forward and up.
- Allow your back to lengthen and widen.

Most of the physical reasons for panic attacks can be traced to over-tensed neck muscles that trigger the fear reflexes (fight or flight response). If we are to obtain a lasting release of muscular tension, the Primary Control should be allowed to work without interference. The Primary Directions help the Primary Control to re-assert itself, and consequently allow the reflexes throughout the body to work as they should, and not to be inappropriately triggered as in the case of panic attacks.

Do not, however, attempt the semi-supine position during a panic attack, as this may cause the adrenaline to stay in your bloodstream for longer and therefore may prolong the length of the attack. Wait until the attack passes.

What to Do If You Have an Attack

During a panic attack the adrenaline that is rushing through your system provides the body with the necessary strength, speed and stamina for survival. In fact, during an attack intense activity such as running on the spot or walking fast may well burn off the adrenaline more quickly. This could decrease the intensity of the attack or shorten its duration. Any exercise that exerts the body and is appropriate for where you are at the time of the attack will do. Also, be aware of how you are moving during any exercise, lest you pull a muscle or tear a ligament. In the unlikely event of an attack coming on when you are lying down, get up immediately and engage yourself in some physical exercise.

Awareness

For one reason or another it may not be possible to be very active during an attack; if this is the case, some other form of distraction may be your best option. Initially, just go into the sensations willingly, because if you try to fight them you will only cause even more tension and may make the situation worse. Be attentive to what is happening to your body - are you, for instance:

- retracting your head backwards?
- hunching your shoulders?

- tensing your jaw?

- clenching your fists?

- arching your back?

- tensing your legs?

- bracing your knees?

- curling your toes up?

Just noticing these sensations may be enough to bring about a change that will help you to come out of the attack, but thinking about the Directions as described in Chapter 2 may help you to release yourself from the vicious cycle of the fear of the attacks and the attacks themselves. Thinking of the Primary and Secondary Directions may be particularly helpful to you during an attack. It is vital, however, that you understand that these Directions need to be learned during your Alexander lessons with a qualified teacher.

Breathing

In times of crisis, placing your attention on your breathing may also help you. Follow your breath as it enters your body; feel the movement of your ribs, abdomen and upper chest as this gentle but powerful occurrence takes place. Just being conscious of the way you breathe may bring about subtle changes which will help you to feel more calm and thus have a neutralizing effect on the panic attack. It is important that you do not force your breathing, either by pushing the breath out or by sucking air in. Natural breathing helps to regulate the levels of oxygen and carbon dioxide in the body, and this in turn can help other bodily functions to work more efficiently.

There has been various research into the effects that the Alexander Technique has on breathing. In the US, Dr John Austin measured both lung capacity and the maximum rate at which people could exhale. Both of these showed a significant improvement after the subjects being studied had a course of Alexander lessons. In The Alexander Technique, author Chris Stevens reports that Dr Wilfred Barlow in the UK and Dr David Galick in Australia independently found that having Alexander lessons was instrumental in slowing down and deepening patterns of breathing. Through Alexander lessons a different pattern of breathing can be obtained which subsequently helps to make the panic attack sufferer more clam and less anxious.

(For more about breathing awareness, see Chapter 8.)

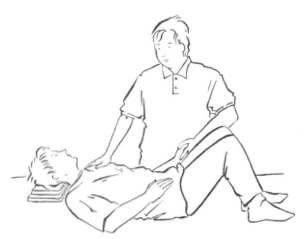

During the first few lessons the Alexander teacher helps the pupil to release tension while lying down

Alexander Lessons

Having Alexander Technique lessons can offer you a real solution to the problems of intense anxiety or panic attacks. One of the fundamental principles behind the Technique is that misuse of the body and mind often occurs habitually and unconsciously (*see Chapter 2*). Put simply, this means that the reason for your anxiety is probably unconscious; you could have deep-rooted concerns of which you are unaware. The Technique is an extremely powerful tool for working directly on the body and mind, and can help to bring your unconsciousness fears and anxieties under control. Even if you suffer from only occasional nervousness, the Technique can be extremely effective in preventing your condition from deteriorating any further.

The results that Alexander lessons can produce are often powerful enough to break the vicious cycle of fear, anxiety and panic in which you may have become trapped. Your Alexander teacher will show you in a practical way how to release muscle tension, and this will allow you to feel calmer and more at ease, both mentally and emotionally. You will eventually feel more in control of the panic and ultimately of yourself.

Your teacher may move your limbs or head gently while asking you *not* to try to help; this is to check for any excessive muscle tension you may be carrying. This may be done while you are standing, sitting or lying on a teaching table. Your teacher will then help you to become aware of the muscular tension that you have been exerting unnecessarily, and will then give you a series of verbal instructions (i.e. the Directions) which will help you to release that tension. Many pupils are surprised when they suddenly become aware of how much tension they are holding in their muscles.

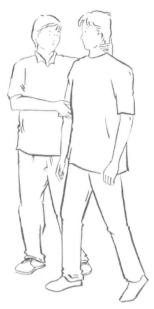

Helping a pupil release tension while walking which allows greater coordination

After a while you may be asked to perform simple actions such as sitting or walking to see if you use any inappropriate physical habits while moving. Some people may be performing such actions with far more muscle tension than they actually need; when they are shown how to carry them out with less effort they feel a lightness and ease in the body that they may not have experienced for many years. You may find yourself talking, eating and acting with less haste, and soon you will be moving with more grace and poise. This feeling of lightness and ease of movement is often described as the hallmark of the Alexander Technique. This feeling occurs as the parts of the body start to work in co-operation with one another instead of, as is frequently the case, against each other. As pupils of the Technique begin to perform actions in new and easier ways, some describe a feeling of 'walking on air' or 'having well-oiled joints'. It is not that you have to learn different actions; it is more a case of ceasing to interfere unconsciously with every movement you make and allowing your body to work as nature intended.

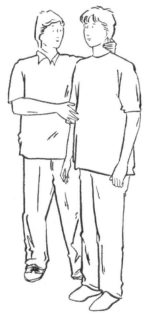

Helping a pupil to achieve a more balanced posture whilst standing

When people who have been suffering from panic attacks first come to me for Alexander lessons, their body can be almost immovable with tension. It does not take very long, however, before they learn how to release the tension and, as they do, the frequency and intensity of their panic attacks lessen. It is often only a matter of weeks before they can really start to see the tremendous benefits that the Technique is making to their lives; they feel, literally and figuratively, as if a great burden had been suddenly lifted from their shoulders.

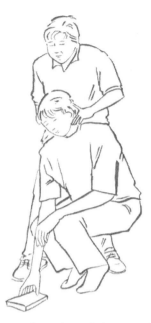

Helping a pupil to achieve balance and coordination while picking up an object

When you first have Alexander lessons, it is important to realize that this sensation may last for only a relatively short time. In fact, after your first lesson the benefits may last for only half an hour or so, but with subsequent lessons the effects will last for longer and longer periods. As your body learns to release the physical tension and your mind and emotions become calmer, you may well find yourself sleeping better, which will give you the rest necessary for a healthy body and peaceful mind. Very soon you will notice the fear and panic steadily moving out of your life and being replaced with a sense of relief and renewed hope as you start to feel your self-confidence and balanced perspective returning.

Eventually, you will be able to apply the principles of the Technique without the aid of a teacher, and gradually you will feel much more relaxed and generally more in control of your life. This process will free you from the fear that creates the attacks in the first place. Try to be patient, because even when you have become more aware of these responses they will not necessarily change immediately. It is important to realize that it takes perseverance, time and practise before you can find the strength and clarity to refuse consistently to react in old, established patterns of behaviour.

If you practise Alexander's principles, eventually you will be able to choose new ways of being and ultimately a new way of life. By practising the Technique you will become much more aware of your habitual responses and reactions in daily life. As you change the way you think and behave you will often find that other people will change in the way they behave towards you.

Hint

The Alexander Technique helps you to release anxiety and to remember how precious this human existence is - it was not given to us to spend in fear.

6
Depression

Use your eyes as if tomorrow you would be stricken blind. And the same method can be applied to other senses. Hear the music of voices, the song of the birds, the mighty strains of an orchestra, as if you would be stricken deaf tomorrow. Touch each object you want to touch as if tomorrow your tactile sense would fail. Smell the perfume of flowers, taste with relish each morsel, as if tomorrow you could never smell and taste again. Make the most of every sense.

Helen Keller

There are many causes of depression. More and more information about the reasons behind it becomes available all the time, but unfortunately scientists and the medical profession seem to be fighting a losing battle as we see the number of people suffering from depression constantly rising. According to the World Health Organization, over 100 million people on our planet are suffering from depression at any one time, and in his article in the Journal of Abnormal Psychology (No 102, 1993), Peter Lewinsohn states that a person born between 1945 and 1954 is 10 times more likely to suffer from depression than someone born between 1905 and 1914. But perhaps the most alarming new evidence to come to light is that the predisposition towards depression is becoming more widespread among the young. Statistics show clearly that with each generation the first bout of depression occurs at an earlier age than in the previous one. Looking at international data, we can see that there seems to be an epidemic of depression.

Effects of Depression

The effects of depression can make it difficult to get out of bed in the morning. Feelings of emptiness, loneliness and loss of energy pervade the sufferer's life. Every movement seems to take more effort than it is worth, and as a result their actions get slower and it takes longer and longer to complete simple daily activities. Even going upstairs or tackling minor chores can be exhausting, and this is mirrored perfectly by the sufferer's listless or slumped posture. Their face also reflects their inner state, becoming expressionless. Emotions are withdrawn and are replaced by a feeling of numbness, guilt and unworthiness.

Acute depression can be one of the worst kinds of affliction, because it taints every part of a person's life and can make them care so little for themselves that they lose the motivation to do anything about their condition - they just can't make themselves carry out even the simplest of actions because they no longer see any point to life. They lose their appetite, and the lack of food then contributes to their already debilitating lack of energy. At its worst, depression may even produce suicidal tendencies.

As with panic attacks and worry, one of the main causes of depression is stress. The symptoms can be similar - fatigue, loss of appetite, erratic sleeping patterns and difficulty in concentrating. Unlike the anxious person, however, the depressed person merely gives up under the strain. The chart below compares anxiety with depression:

Depression	Anxiety
Feelings of emptiness, lethargy or desolation	Feelings of worry, apprehension, unease or fear
Body pulled down with tension, causing a slumped posture	Body rigid with tension
Body movements slow; everything is an effort	Speeding up of body movements until actions are jerky or erratic
Often blame themselves for their problems, and can be plagued by feelings of guilt or worthlessness	Often blame others for their problems
Feel worse in the mornings and find it hard to get motivated	Find it hard to wind down and generally feel worse in the evenings
Loss of interest in everything and lacking ambition	Over-anxiety about obtaining results
Slowing down of thoughts	Speeding up of thoughts

Causes of Depression

There are many theories and hypotheses about the causes of depression, but to simplify matters they can be separated into five major categories:

1. Physical
2. Behavioural
3. Psychological
4. Reactive
5. Chemical

Physical

The way we use our bodies can contribute to or may even cause depressive feelings; over many years, a person's poor posture and way of holding themselves can become ingrained to such an extent that their movements can start to feel sluggish. We all know how exercise can contribute to feelings of well-being. People who feel almost continually lethargic will experience increasingly negative thoughts about life. Physical sluggishness of this kind can be exacerbated by long hours of sitting at a desk, especially on badly designed furniture, by long hours in a car or as a result of any repetitive occupation where one has to stay in one place for long periods. It can also be a 'learned' trait copied in childhood from our parents or peers.

Behavioural

As children, a majority of the things we learn take place by copying those around us. The way we behave can be influence by the habits of our close family; even as children we begin to take on the characteristics of our parents, which become reinforced in adulthood. It is easy for people outside the family to see the uncanny similarities, but those on the inside are often oblivious to these 'family traits'. Is it not possible that some cases of depression that are supposed to be hereditary could simply be due to the fact that we have copied the emotional habits of our parents?

Psychological

Events in early childhood may have a profound effect on emotional development. Problems could be caused, for example, by an unloving or unaffectionate parent, or by being sent away to boarding school at an early age. Low self-esteem is a hallmark of depression.

A person can also suffer from depression because they have been taught inappropriate and unnatural responses to certain situations while young. For example, if someone has been taught that getting angry or expressing sadness is not acceptable, or is even wrong, they may have extreme difficulty in exhibiting these emotions in their adult life. It has been written that depression is anger turned inwards. Unexpressed sorrow can also result in depression.

Reactive

Events that may cause the onset of depression can be loss of a family member or close friend, divorce or separation, disharmonious home life, unemployment, stagnation and boredom, or generally feeling trapped and as if we have no choice about our career, lifestyle or relationships.

Chemical

Medical doctors often suggest that depression is caused by a hormonal or chemical imbalance, which may have a genetic cause. Although this information has been very useful and has helped some people who suffer from endogenous depression, it has caused others to think that they are victims of circumstance and that there is little they can do about their plight. Even when the reason for depression is an imbalance of the body's chemical make-up, is it not possible that this may be due to the continual release of hormones which occurs during prolonged periods of stress?

Posture and Depression

Whatever the cause, one way that depression reveals itself in the sufferer is the way they hold their body. They invariably sit or stand in a slumped fashion and are rarely interested in what is going on around them. It is even of note that we describe this mental and emotional condition in physical terms - to depress means to press down. If the body, mind and emotions are inseparable, as Alexander claimed, then unless the use of the body is improved, the depressed person will have little hope of escaping their predicament. This improvement can happen directly or indirectly:

- Directly: by working on the body to improve posture, poise and the general way we move during the performance of everyday tasks
- Indirectly: by changing the way we react to emotional problems or by altering our perception of external circumstances.

In my experience, if a person who suffers from depression improves their posture by using the Alexander Technique, their depression often lifts and they become more interested in life generally. In my opinion, unless a person learns to use themselves in an improved way then the chances of their depression recurring after established forms of treatment will be very high. This partly explains why some people can have psychotherapy for many years with little success: it is not that the psychotherapy is, in itself, ineffectual, but rather that little progress can be made unless the person also changes on a physical level.

Hint

If we are ever to find a solution to this growing problem of depression, we must not forget the immortal words of Plato: "The cure of the part should not be attempted without the treatment of the whole."

Overcoming Depression

The hardest thing you need to do is to be determined continually to beat the habit of depression. It is often the last thing you are going to feel capable of, but deal with it you must. To overcome your feelings of depression you will have to change emotionally, mentally and physically. You will have to take risks - in exposing your feelings, in expressing your innermost thoughts and in being who you are, even though all your past conditioning may have taught you the opposite:

To laugh is to risk appearing a fool,

To weep is to risk appearing sentimental,

To reach out for another is to risk involvement,

To expose your feelings is to risk rejection,

To place your dreams before a crowd is to risk ridicule,

To love is to risk not being loved in return.

To go forward in the face of overwhelming odds is to risk failure.

But risks must be taken because the real hazard in life is to risk nothing,

The person who risks nothing does nothing, has nothing, is nothing,

He may avoid suffering and sorrow, but he cannot learn to feel, change, love or grow,

Chained by his certitudes, he is a slave, he has forfeited his freedom.

Only the person who has the courage to take risks is free.

Anon

It may help you to talk openly about your feelings, especially when you feel depression looming. It is important for you to realize that other people do not have to give you a solution to your problems: merely acknowledging and talking about your feelings can help to open your mind to positive thoughts rather than negative ones.

Reactive Depression

Even with reactive depression it is not necessarily the events in life that bring on the illness; it is the way we view, and consequently react to, these events. Two people with similar problems or tension in their lives can react in completely different ways: one seeing it as a challenge, the other as overwhelming pressure. You may think '*if only* things had been different I would be happy,' but this kind of mindset will forever hold you back from dealing with your life as it is now; you will instead waste valuable energy dwelling on what might have been.

Exercise

Rather than let your mind wander on to negative trains of thought, try constantly to bring it back to the present moment. To achieve this, you could begin to notice the colours, shapes and textures of objects around you, or while walking down a familiar street try to spot things that you have never noticed before. Even if you find this difficult at first, don't give up; by persevering, you will start to become aware of many things you have never noticed - perhaps the movement or sound caused by the wind in the trees; the shape of windows or the roofs on the houses; the feeling of the sun, rain or wind on your face, or even the way you are standing or walking. All these things will help you to engage with your environment and ultimately help you to live in the present.

Tip

Remember that your wandering mind and negative thoughts are your greatest enemy. They will age you before your time - do not enter into allegiance with them. The words in the poem Living Forces by General MacArthur may help give you the courage and inspiration you need to beat your depression, and in so doing to rediscover your natural enthusiasm for life.

Youth is not a stage in life,
it is a condition of the spirit,
a result of will, an intensity of emotion,
a victory of courage over timidity,
of the taste of adventure over the love of physical comfort.
One does not become old by living for a certain number of years,
one becomes old because one has left behind one's ideals. Years
wrinkle the skin, but to renounce one's ideals wrinkles the soul.
Preoccupation, doubts, worries and loss of hope are the enemies
which slowly incline us towards the ground, so that we become dust
before our death.
A person is young when they know how to be awe-struck by life.
That person is inquisitive, like the insatiable child. They defy life's
difficult events and find joy in the game of life.
You are as old as your faith, or as old as your doubt.
As young as your confidence in yourself, as young as your hope, as

old as your submission.

You will stay young as long as you are open and receptive;
receptive to all that is beautiful, good and great,
 receptive to nature's messages of humanity and the infinite.
 If one day your heart would be bitten by pessimism and gnawed
by cynicism; then may God have mercy upon your soul that has
grown old.

These are strong words, but you need strength if you are ever to break the chains of depression that leave you feeling stagnant and dejected and prevent you from enjoying you life to the full.

Depression and Alexander's Directions

Over-tensed back muscles interfere with the freedom of the Primary Control (the dynamic relationship of the head to the neck and spine). Giving yourself 'Directions' is the process whereby an improved posture and way of movement can be obtained. This will automatically change the way you think and feel about yourself.

The following Directions can be especially helpful to those who are suffering from depression. However, it is important to realize that they should be combined with Inhibition and the Primary Directions (*see Chapter 2*), as these directly help the Primary Control to return to its natural state of freedom, and consequently encourage the reflexes and muscle throughout the body to work appropriately.

Secondary Directions that Can Help Depression

- *Allow your shoulders to release away from one another.* This will help to achieve release across the upper chest, very beneficial to anyone with rounded shoulders - a common tendency in those who suffer from depression.

- *Allow your left shoulder to release away from your right hip, and your right shoulder to release away from your left hip.* It is very common for people who suffer from depression to pull down with the muscles in the front of the body. This Direction can be very helpful in releasing the tension in these muscles.

- *Think of allowing your hands to widen as your fingers lengthen.* This can help anyone who unconsciously clenches their fists when under stress.

- *Think of not pushing your pelvis forward.* This can prevent over-arching of the back - the common habit of depression sufferers as they try to straighten themselves out of their 'pulled down' posture.

- *Think of not bracing your knees back.* This can be effective in releasing tension in the legs, which again is very common in those who have poor posture caused by depression. Be careful that you do not over-compensate by standing with your knees bent.

- *Think of your feet spreading on to the ground as your toes lengthen.* This can release tension in the toes and will help you to walk more easily and feel more balanced.

These are some of the most relevant Secondary Directions. After a number of Alexander lessons you will be able to give yourself these Directions during your everyday activities. Practising these Directions may also help to free the rib cage and improve your breathing (*also see Chapter 8*).

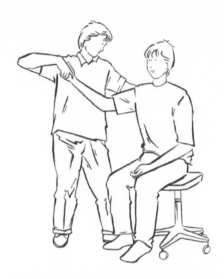

Releasing the tension that has been pulling you down will help you to feel lighter; since the body, mind and emotions are interconnected, you may start to develop a less bleak, more positive outlook on life as a result

Getting Help

Initially, you will need the help of an Alexander Technique teacher who will show you how to improve your posture and move more freely. During your lessons, your teacher may suggest you try other Directions pertinent to your particular condition.

As we saw earlier, Alexander realized that he could not change the way he used his body merely by 'doing' something, as that actually created an increase in tension. In the same way, if you suffer from depression it is no use just 'standing up straight' or 'getting your shoulders back': you will have to release the tension in the muscles that have been pulling you down in the first place. If you merely make an effort to change your 'depressed' posture, the new muscle tension will simply be pulling in the opposite direction to the original tension. The net effect is that you are likely to give up after a short time as you will not be able to sustain the tremendous effort which is needed. If you are ever to release the tension associated depression effectively you will need to do less rather than more. This is why just thinking of the Directions can be so effective.

It is widely believed that we are accountable for what we do, but not for what we think. In truth we are responsible for both our thoughts and our actions. What we do arises from how we think. As already explained, the way we use our minds causes the tension that leads to muscle contraction and causes us to depress our bodies into the slumped shape that invariably accompanies mental depression. In direct contrast, during Alexander lessons the body lengthens and widens as a result of releasing tension. At first many people think that Alexander simply devised a relaxation technique - by using Directions your body *can* become less tense or rigid, but this does not mean that you allow your limbs to go completely slack or limp. Instead, the body attains a state of 'relaxed alertness' similar to that of a domestic cat.

By learning to release unnecessary tension, you will stop interfering with the body's natural balance and co-ordination mechanisms and reflexes. As a result, your body will automatically lengthen and widen, allowing you to experience a new sense of freedom and peace. These inspiring words from George Bernard Shaw, one of Alexander's personal pupils, may help those who suffer from depression to find a way to conquer their problem:

*People are always blaming circumstances for what they are. I do
not believe in circumstances. The people who get on in this world
are the people who get up and look for the circumstances they want,
and if they cannot find them, make them.*

When you change your circumstances by means of Inhibition and creative thought, then you will be practising the Alexander Technique.

Important Note

If you are suffering from clinical depression it is vital to consult your doctor in conjunction with having Alexander lessons. If you have been prescribed medication for your depression, do not stop taking it without the advice and supervision of your doctor.

7
Stress and Emotions

Anyone can become angry - that is easy. But to be
angry with the right person, to the right degree, at the
right time, for the right purpose, and in the right way
- this is not easy.

Aristotle

Stress strikes at the heart of our emotional world and undermines
our relationships and the social fabric as a whole.

Family Disintegration

One of the main reasons why relationships become strained is that
people today generally do not have time to nourish them. We may
think that by 'stressing ourselves out' we will be thought of as responsible, but as Stuart Wilde points out in his little book of common
sense entitled Life Was Never Meant to Be a Struggle:

If I bust a gut and hurtle around and try hard, people will see me
as a good man and they will treat me with respect. Whether I get
results or not matters little, as long as I am seen to be making a
valiant effort. To make sure everyone acknowledges my heroism I
will create an entire theatre of frantic action, hectic schedules, long
hours and constant pressure. Of course, this pantomime will make

me a bit tense, but that is all part of the act. For the tension will be
seen by others as my taking responsibility and they will love and
respect me for that. Won't they?

He goes on to say that if the truth be known, the answer is *no*! And in fact, this person's lack of self-esteem stands out a mile and his frantic actions serve only to underline that he is out of control and does not really have a clue what he is doing.

The irony is that the more stressed we are, the more we need the support of family. But if we cannot take the time and trouble to nurture our relationships with those closest to us, how can we expect them to be there for us when we need them?

If we stop for a moment and use our common sense, we can see that in our endeavour to be seen to be responsible and to be respected and loved, we risk losing everything we hold dear - our own family and the enjoyment of life itself.

Unemployment

We are living in uncertain times where fewer and fewer people have the security of long-term employment. Even after faithfully working long hours over a number of years, many people have found themselves unemployed. Because of the stigma that is placed on the unemployed and the fact that our identity often becomes tied up with the work we do, many people are unable to cope with being made redundant. It is ironic that many of those in work yearn for the weekends, holidays or retirement, while those out of work can't wait to get a job, and there seems to be an ever-increasing imbalance between those who have too much work to do and those who have no work at all. Like the overworked person, the unemployed person can suffer from stress or low self-esteem and may struggle for many years with feelings of inadequacy. In both cases, the stress occurs because life is not as they would wish. The way to reduce this stress, whatever the external circumstance, is to remove the erroneous ideas and conditioning about our self-worth being tied up with what we do for a living; we are important simply because we are human beings.

Appreciation

When two people first meet and fall in love, even if they have busy work schedules they both make sure that they spend quality time with each other which makes each of them feel loved and appreciated. Over time, however, work and other commitments begin to hold sway and unconscious habits of stress are set up within the relationship. The undeniable pressure that they are under can cause them to feel exhausted and they therefore have little left to give to each other at the end of the day. This can be especially true of women, who even in this age of supposed equality have to cope with looking after the children and many of the domestic chores as well as full-time employment. Overwork, constant tiredness and the resulting irritability are the perfect recipe for a disastrous relationship.

If this situation is allowed to continue for a period of time it may cause people to express their anger at not being loved or appreciated. Critical remarks, arguments, fights or even violence may erupt. This kind of behaviour eventually becomes the norm, the two people involved finding it hard to break the habit even when they want to. Eventually they may seek solace and recognition in another love affair, which for a short time may help to restore their self-esteem, but in the long term the cycle is likely to repeat itself. Each time we return to the point where we feel trapped, unloved or stagnant, we lose even more confidence in ourselves and gradually begin to lose all faith and trust in life.

Whatever stage you are at in your relationship, you can improve it by taking steps to remove the external circumstances which cause stress. The realization that your partner is feeling just as stressed as you can help you to see that the way forward is not to argue about it, but to work together to combat it. Since the Alexander Technique helps you to break habits by becoming more conscious of them, it can be helpful when emotional issues such as these arise in your life.

Uncontrollable Emotions

Constant stress in a person's life will frequently trigger emotional distress which can soon become overwhelming.

High emotion takes a significant physical toll: the heart rate can increase by 10, 20 or even 30 beats a minute, muscles become even tenser than usual and breathing becomes more rapid.

In his book Emotional Intelligence, Daniel Goleman describes the experience of these uncontrolled emotions clearly:

There is a swamp of toxic feelings, an unpleasant wash of fear and anger that seem inescapable and, subjectively, takes 'forever' to get over. At this point a person's emotions are so intense, their perspective so narrow, and their thinking so confused that there is no hope of taking the other's viewpoint or settling things in a reasonable way.

When a person is on 'the receiving end' of such outbursts, Goleman explains that he or she starts to be 'on guard' for the next emotional assault or injustice, becoming habitually hypervigilant for any sign of attack, insult or grievance, and bound to over-react at even the slightest sign. This defensive behaviour against personal criticism merely adds fuel to the fire, and the original source of tension between the two parties becomes more deeply entrenched, leading to further outbursts of uncontrollable emotion.

Traditionally, men are taught not to 'succumb' to their emotions; instead they 'shut down' emotionally in the face of grief or anger. In some instances this may represent an effective safety mechanism, as it has been shown, for example, that men who are easily roused to anger are three times more likely to die of cardiac arrest as those who are more even-tempered. It may not be the anger itself that increases the risk of heart disease, but rather that tense situations frequently send a rush of stress hormones around the body. The problem is, however, that if in the midst of an argument with his wife the husband 'cuts off' from any emotional interaction, this causes his wife's heart rate shoots up. In the long term his emotional distance limits his capacity to engage fully with other human beings, and exacerbates the emotional stress felt by the women in his life.

Emotional Inhibition

The starting point in resolving emotional problems is to stand back and analyse the underlying cause of the difficulties we may be experiencing. In other words, the same *Inhibition* that allows us to make choices while performing our daily actions is also required in order to change the way we react emotionally.

It is far more difficult to practise Inhibition when it comes to emotional issues, because by their very nature they can seem 'beyond our control'. Their roots may extend far back into past experiences and be buried deep in our subconscious. Various 'triggers' may allow this past or hidden pain to come to the surface. This is why apparently small issues in our relationships with others may spark off a major argument. Without Inhibition, we run among other risks that of giving voice to criticisms that can only cause more damage and fuel our own fear of being unloved and unlovable.

Being able to inhibit emotions is no easy task; plenty of practice is needed to perfect the art. We must first learn to apply Inhibition to simple everyday actions; once we have mastered this we can use it in more volatile situations.

Remember that Inhibition is not the suppression of emotion: it is the chance to pause in order to turn potentially emotionally destructive situations into constructive ones. Inhibition helps you to be more patient and understanding of others' emotional feelings as well as your own.

This Hopi Native American saying reflects how Inhibition can be useful during situations involving conflict:

Take care
when you speak in judgement.
Words are powerful weapons
which can cause many tragedies.
Never make a person look like a fool with your tongue.
Never make a person look small with your big mouth.
A hard word, a sharp word,
can burn a long time,
deep in the heart,
leaving a scar.
Accept that others
think differently,

act differently,

feel differently,

speak differently.

Be mild and healing with your words.

Words should be lights!

Words should be calm.

Bring people together,

Bring peace.

Where words are weapons,

people face each other

like enemies.

Life is much too short and our world is much too tiny

to turn it into a battlefield.

By using the Alexander Technique, it is possible to express emotions without letting them get out of control, and to acquire the patience to hear others out before you jump in with your own point of view. Inhibition and Direction can be very helpful in resolving conflict, enabling you to have conscious control in a situation that requires calm and collected behaviour without suppressing feelings.

Emotional Restraint and Children

When dealing with children's emotions, the same kind of restraint is required. If we are able to hold back and assess the situation before taking action, then our children will learn this skill as well.

When a child accidentally spills a drink, under normal circumstances we would not get upset and would reassure the child that accidents happen to everyone. If we are under stress, however, we may become irritable and can find ourselves shouting angrily at the child. Children can become confused by such mixed messages and inconsistencies in our behaviour. Obviously, children need guidelines, but if these are constantly changing depending on our moods then they are going to find it difficult to work out what is the appropriate response to a given event. Children are often extremely intuitive and know instinctively when they are being treated unfairly; the greater the restrictions placed upon them while they are young, the more they may rebel when they reach their teenage years.

Children can often be the innocent victims of stress and can mistakenly think that they are to blame for the unsettled atmosphere at home. They can become bewildered and frightened by arguments or periods of tense silence between their parents. Inhibition can help you to deal not only with your own emotions but with those of your children, and can help you to show them by example the calm and peace that can be obtained by handling emotion from a position of calm and thoughtfulness.

Taking Responsibility

Sometimes it seems that there are so many problems, emotional and otherwise, that it is almost impossible to know where to start trying to solve them. Some people hope that with a change of government things might get better, others look to their doctor for an answer in the form of the latest stress-combating drug. Yet you bear the ultimate responsibility for the quality of your life; no one else can enrich it for you. You are the only one who can make the improvements necessary to calm your emotions, clear your mind and improve your physical well-being.

The way we improve the quality of life is simple. It does not cost us money, nor time. Attention is all it takes. The Alexander Technique enables us to be more conscious so that we can realize our true and wonderful potential. The price of being unconscious is pain - be it physical pain, mental torment or emotional turmoil, but the rewards and joy that accompany a conscious life are very desirable.

> *If there be righteousness in the heart,*
> *there will be beauty in the character.*
> *If there be beauty in the character,*
> *there will be harmony in the home.*
> *If there be harmony in the home,*
> *there will be order in the nation.*
> *If there be order in the nation,*
> *there will be peace in the world.*

By using the Alexander Technique we can become more conscious of how we react in different situations and will be able to cultivate the ability to 'stand back' when emotions are in danger of running away with us. This can help to dissolve conflict more quickly, and with less harmful results. This does not mean becoming emotionally distant or detached, but cultivating the ability to listen actively to what others have to say, with interest and compassion.

Faulty Perception

Another reason to use Inhibition is so that you have time to consider the validity of your point of view. We all make mistakes sometimes - this is a natural part of being human - but many of us confuse being *right* with being a *success*, while being *wrong* equals *failure*. We rarely consider for a moment that we might be wrong, because we have come to learn that backing down and admitting our mistakes is humiliating or embarrassing.

> Alexander told his pupils not to come to him unless they were pleased when he told them that they were wrong.

Most of the information that we retain in our brain we have had to learn at some stage in life *from someone else* - who is to say that this information is always correct? Maybe it is worth considering this saying from the Talmud:

We do not see things as they are.
We see them as we are.

Inhibition gives us the time and opportunity to check that our thoughts and feelings regarding a person, experience or situation are *still relevant and correct for us as we are now.*

Expressing Gratitude

One of the most noticeable results that students of the Alexander Technique achieve is that they begin to feel that they have more time to give to their families simply, because they are no longer preoccupied with their own problems. As their muscle tension is released, they feel more optimistic about life and generally more cheerful. In short, they are better company. Uncomfortable feelings such as mood swings, irritability, gloom, anger or even rage are replaced with a new sense of calm, light-heartedness and easy-goingness. They feel transformed as they shed their old behavioural patterns that caused them so much emotional imbalance.

Being a more conscious human being allows you to be aware of many of life's small pleasures, and as a result you may be more able to feel gratitude in your life. This will naturally be taken into your emotional life, and these feelings of appreciation will be reciprocated by your family, friends and colleagues at work. After 10 lessons I often ask my pupils what effects they have experienced, and whatever reason they originally came for, nearly all of them say that they are feeling happier. During my time as an Alexander Technique teacher I have also seen a number of marriages saved by the change of attitude undergone by my students. The partners of these students have commented time and time again on the remarkable change they have witnessed, and after a course of lessons they say that their partner is a much nicer person to live with. By living more consciously, you will be able to value the people with whom you share your life. I often think of these words by Anna Cummins:

> Do not save your loving speeches
> For your friends till they are dead;
> Do not write them on their tombstones,
> Speak them rather now instead.

By being more conscious, you will be able to express appreciation to those around you and this can lead to a happier, more harmonious life. Please do not think that you will be able to do this overnight; as you will have understood by now, Inhibition and Direction take time to master before you will be able to reap the benefits of a calmer and more balanced emotional life.

8
The Breath
of Life

The same stream of life that runs through my veins
night and day runs through the world and dances in
rhythmic measures.

It is the same life that shouts in joy through the dust
of the Earth in numberless blades of grass and breaks
into tumultuous waves of leaves and flowers.

It is the same life that rocked in the ocean cradle of
birth and of death, in ebb and in flow.

I feel my limbs are made glorious by the touch of this
world of life and my pride is from life, the throb of
ages dancing in my blood this moment.

Rahbindranath Tagore

Our breath quietly and consistently rises and falls during every moment of our existence; it was the first action we performed as we entered this life and it will surely be the last before we die; its gentle presence is there with us through the happy times as well as in our darkest hour; it is the one thing that is common to every single one of us, no matter what race, sex, colour or religion we are. It is our very essence, and connects us to the creative force that is responsible for everything that we experience around us. Yet for all this, for the most part it goes unnoticed and unappreciated.

This is not new information - everyone *knows* that if we stop breathing we die in a matter of minutes, yet how many of us take a moment to *realize* how precious each breath really is? We are far more inclined to take it all for granted, but without each and every breath nothing else would have any importance whatsoever; we would not exist.

Without breath we could not utter a single word or perform even the smallest of actions. The life-force itself automatically causes us to take a breath without any effort on our part; we do not even have to remember to breathe. Saint Augustine once said that people travel to wonder at the heights of mountains, at the huge waves of the sea, at the long courses of rivers, at the vast compass of the ocean, at the circular motion of the stars; and all too often they pass by themselves without wondering at all.

Tip

Just pause for a moment as you are reading these words to become aware of that silent inhalation and exhalation which is with you every moment of your life. Without it, you would not be able to see these words, hear the sound of the pages as they turn, feel the texture of the paper, or even move one muscle to hold this book. Contemplate the mysteries of your breath and see if you can get a sense of what force or energy is drawing the air into and then out of your lungs.

Posture and Breathing

Efficient and beneficial breathing is an integral part of good posture and a clear mind, and generally using the body in the way it was designed to be used. Like many other functions of the body, this simple act of breathing is often unconsciously interfered with. As we have seen, poor posture and misuse of the body can cause an over-tensing of the entire muscular system; this can affect the functioning of the ribcage, the lungs, and even the nasal passage, mouth and throat (trachea) through which air passes. Muscle tension can also produce a general 'collapsing' or slumping of the torso, which can result in a massive restriction in the lungs' capacity to take in air, leading to shallow breathing. In short, if we use our body incorrectly we can make the effortless act of breathing hard work.

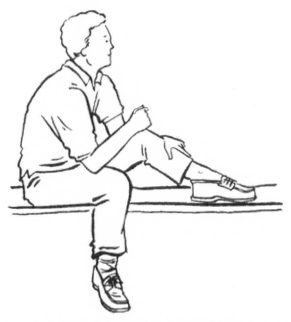

Examples of slumped and twisted postures

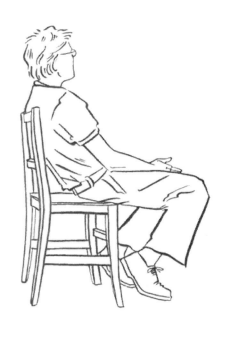

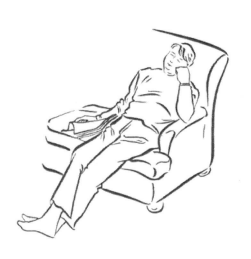

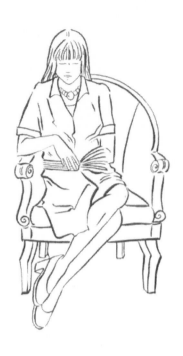

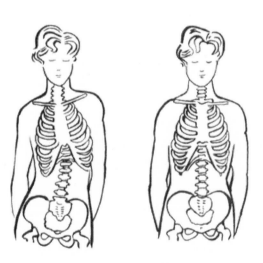

A twisted posture puts strain on the spine and affects breathing

Interference with the respiratory system can sometimes be traced back to early childhood, or even to the first few days of life if the shock of birth was traumatic, but it usually starts around the age of five or six. It is at this age that we are first forced to hold certain 'set' positions for long periods of time. Poor posture is often the result, making our movements ungraceful, uncoordinated or even clumsy, and restricting our breathing patterns.

These detrimental respiratory habits may go unnoticed during childhood or adolescence, but the effects of shallow breathing can be seen in adulthood as they become more accentuated. In severe cases, it is possible to observe adults unnecessarily raising and lowering their shoulders while inhaling and exhaling, while others fix the ribcage, hold their abdominal muscles rigid and then lift and collapse the chest in order just to breathe. By comparison, if you observe a baby or young child you may notice how much their abdomen and ribcage move in and out rhythmically with each breath. The rest of the body remains in a state of relaxation.

Tip

It is essential to understand that you need to do *less* in order for your natural way of breathing to return.

If your body is unable to get enough oxygen because its natural deeper breathing is being interfered with, it will have to find another way of achieving this objective. In order to get the oxygen it requires, the breathing rate will have to be increased and as a result a quicker, more shallow type of respiration occurs. Severe restriction of the functioning of the respiratory system will also affect all the other systems of the body, as each one needs sufficient oxygen in order to function efficiently.

Stress and Breathing

Shallow breathing can also cause or exacerbate anxiety, worry, panic attacks and depression; in turn, all these conditions are likely to cause interference with the breathing mechanism, so it is sometimes difficult to know 'which came first': did the emotional state trigger the breathing problems, or vice versa? Physical, mental and emotional conditions are so intrinsically linked to one another that it is best to consider them as inseparable.

By applying the Alexander Technique to the action of breathing we can become aware of the detrimental habits which interfere with this delicate process, and can relearn our natural rhythm of breathing. As a consequence, we can alter the way we think, feel and act while carrying out our everyday activities.

I find that when people first come for lessons, even when they do not specifically complain of asthma or other respiratory problems, their breathing is often very erratic or too fast, and they do not even give themselves time to finish one breath before they start the next. This is a direct reflection of how they have been living their lives, and they will frequently say that they feel that there are never enough hours in the day. After a course of Alexander lessons I have found that the breathing rate of these students has been greatly reduced, by up to a third of what it was at first.

Breathing Awareness

Many voice trainers and physical educators encourage 'deep breathing' as a way of getting the lungs to work as they should. While their aim may be sound in principle, the way they encourage their students to achieve this may actually exacerbate many respiratory problems.

People are often instructed to increase their lung capacity by 'pulling in' or 'pushing out' their breath, but this only further tenses an already over-strained muscular system. Almost all breathing techniques focus on the in-breath, as for example the instruction to 'take a deep breath', but this will invariably cause the person to interfere actively with the breathing mechanisms even further. Arching the back and lifting the chest actually restrict breathing, causing additional breathing patterns or ingraining the original breathing habits even more deeply.

Like the rest of the Alexander Technique, breathing naturally is a process of *un-learning* detrimental habits rather than practising certain breathing techniques. Dr Wilfred Barlow, a well-known Alexander teacher and consultant rheumatologist in the British National Health Service, was convinced that people with asthma need 'breathing education' rather than a set of exercises. In his book *The Alexander Principle*, he says:

> *Breathing exercises have, of course, frequently been given by physiotherapists for this and for other breathing conditions, but the fact is that breathing exercises do not help the asthmatic greatly - in fact, recent studies show that after a course of 'breathing exercises', the majority of people breathe less efficiently than they did before they started them.*

Improving Breathing

Alexander was a trained actor and efficient breathing was essential to his skilful recitation. His Technique is based on 'doing less' and stopping interfering with the breathing. One of his most famous quotations was 'I see at last that if I don't breathe … I breathe,' and while still teaching in Australia he was nicknamed 'the breathing man.' When performing, many actors and musicians become nervous, and this tension adversely affects their performance or may even prevent them from performing altogether. In the same way, when we suffer from anxiety or stress our breathing is immediately affected. By ensuring that we breathe naturally, we can effectively combat the effects of stress. In this way, we will feel calmer and more in control even at times of intense emotional or mental tension.

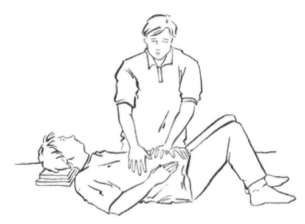

By releasing tension around the rib cage, breathing naturally becomes deeper and slower; as a result, the person will feel calmer

The first thing to do to improve your breathing is simply to become aware of the breath without trying to change it. Just placing your attention on how you breathe may bring about an improvement. Take a moment to lie down and begin to be aware of your breathing - it is often easier to detect tension in this position. Ask yourself the following questions:

- How rapid is my breathing?

- How deeply do I breathe?

- Are my ribs moving as I breathe?

- How much movement is there in the abdominal region when I breathe?

- Do I feel any restriction in my breathing, and if so, where?

It is *vital* that you *do not deliberately change* the way you breathe and that you simply become *aware* of the inhalation and the exhalation, as this is enough to bring about a favourable change. By detecting tension and then releasing it you will start to breathe naturally.

Contrary to what many people think, it is the out-breath, rather than the in-breath, that determines the way we breathe; as we exhale the atmospheric pressure in our lungs decreases, creating a partial vacuum which causes the air from outside to be sucked into our lungs *without us having to do anything*. Under normal conditions the entire breathing mechanism should be self-governing and therefore is sometimes referred to as working 'autonomically'. The more carbon dioxide we exhale, the deeper the next inhalation will be and the deeper our breathing will become. To help his pupils relearn how to breathe naturally, Alexander developed the following method, which is known as 'the whispered ah procedure'. He always maintained that he did not like using exercises as they could encourage bad habits and often stopped people thinking for themselves, but he made an exception for the following procedure because he maintained that it was essentially an exercise in Inhibition and would prevent 'end-gaining' while breathing.

The 'Whispered Ah' Procedure

1. First notice where your tongue is and let it rest on the floor of your mouth, the tip lightly touching your lower front teeth. This allows for a free passage of air to and from the lungs.

2. Make sure your lips and facial muscles are not tense. To assist in this, it may be helpful to *think* of something that makes you smile.

3. Gently and *without straining*, let your lower jaw drop so that your mouth is open. If you allow gravity to do most of the work you will make sure that your head does not tilt backwards in the process.

4. *Whisper* an 'ah' sound (as in the word father) until you come to the natural end of the breath. It is important not to rush the procedure by forcing the air out too quickly or trying to empty the lungs by extending the 'ah' sound for too long.

5. Gently close your lips and *allow* the air to come in through your nose and fill up your lungs.

6. Repeat this procedure several times.

Be aware of your breath as it travels in through your nose, down your throat and into your lungs. Just being conscious of your breathing will bring about subtle changes of which you may not even be aware. Again, it is important to remember that *trying* to change your breathing in any way will interfere with the body's natural processes.

On inhalation, the air has to travel through the bridge of your nose; it might be helpful to *imagine* that you are breathing in through your eyes, as this will prevent tightening of your neck or throat muscles during this procedure.

Regular practice of the 'whispered ah' will help you to notice detrimental breathing habits and eventually to develop a more efficient respiratory system. Once again, it is strongly recommended that initially you go through this routine with an Alexander teacher. This is because most of us suffer from what, as mentioned earlier, Alexander termed *faulty sensory appreciation*, which simply means that even when we are following instructions to the best of our ability we may be doing something else entirely without realizing it. For example, it is very common for people to pull their head back rather than let the jaw drop while carrying out the third instruction, while others are convinced that they are opening their mouth wide when there is actually less than two centimetres between their upper and lower lips. If for any reason you are unable to have lessons (for instance, because that there is no teacher near you), then it is advisable to perform the 'whispered ah' in front of a mirror as this will give you some idea of whether or not you are carrying out the instructions correctly.

Tip

It is essential to understand that the respiratory mechanism works by reflex and is therefore completely automatic. Anything we *do* in order to improve our breathing will only interfere with it further. We need to 'get out of the way' and let nature take its course.

The Enjoyment of Breathing

Not only is breathing an essential part of existence, but natural breathing can be one of life's great joys. It can be a pure pleasure to feel the air filling you with life and offering you the gift of yet another moment to appreciate life's wonders. Being aware of your breathing and practising the 'whispered ah' regularly can be a powerful way to eliminate the effects of stress, as it calms your entire system and allows you to return to the present moment to experience the true miracle of being alive.

By *allowing* your breathing to become more natural it will also become deeper and freer, and your body will start to function more efficiently. Many people experience a feeling of being 'energized' with renewed enthusiasm for life as they feel the power of their spirit flowing through them. With every breath comes another opportunity to throw away the habits that bind us so tightly and start to make real choices. Through free choice we have the power to turn life into what we want it to be.

9
The Freedom
to Change

The snow goose need not bathe
to make itself white.
Neither need you do anything
but be yourself.

Lao Tse

Today there are many people offering a multitude of solutions for reducing stress. Some say that the answer lies in physical exercises - hatha yoga, working out in the gym, jogging, aerobics, swimming, competitive sport or even just going for a long walk. Others proclaim that relaxation method such as meditation, more frequent holidays or simply putting your feet up will help. A third group may even tell you to have psychotherapy so that you can scream or hit a cushion to release the pent-up anger that may be at the root of your muscle tension.

How many of these solutions actually work? Indeed, your first impression of the Alexander Technique may be that it is just the latest in the never-ending series of fads claiming to have the answers to all your problems. It is, in fact, something very different.

First off, the Technique is not new: it has been with us for more than a century. Secondly, it has now achieved worldwide recognition and is being taught by thousands of Alexander teachers in such diverse countries such as Argentina, New Zealand, Malaysia, India and Sweden. Thirdly, over the years the Alexander Technique has gained the approval of many scientific and medical professionals who have spoken with high regard for Alexander and his principles, such as those quoted in this chapter.

Influential Testimonies

Over the years a number of distinguished people have benefited greatly from the Alexander Technique; these include John Cleese, Roald Dahl, Kevin Kline, Edna O'Brien, Paul Newman, Sting and Paul and Linda McCartney, to name but a few. The writer Aldous Huxley was another who was so impressed with the Technique that in his novel *Eyeless in Gaza* he based the character of Miller on Alexander. Huxley sought help from Alexander personally because he was suffering from acute exhaustion and depression; at the time of his first lesson he was only able to write while lying on his back with a typewriter on his chest. After having daily lessons from Alexander, Huxley's general health soon improved and it was not long before he was making public appearances again. He had this to say about his experience of the Technique:

It is now possible to conceive of a totally new type of education affecting the entire range of human activity, from the physiological, through the intellectual, moral, and practical, to the spiritual - an education which by teaching them the proper use of the self, would preserve children and adults from most of the diseases and evil habits that now afflict them; an education whose training in inhibition and conscious control would provide men and women with the psycho-physical means for behaving rationally and morally.

The playwright George Bernard Shaw was another of Alexander's loyal supporters. Shaw approached Alexander at the age of 80, seeking relief from angina. He benefited immediately from the lessons, and lived on to the ripe old age of 94.

Edward Maisel, Director of American Fitness Research and consultant to the President's Council on Physical Fitness, also found lessons in the Alexander Technique extremely effective. In his book *The Resurrection of the Body*, he described the benefits of these lessons:

> *There are an overall flexibility and tonic ease of movement, greater freedom in the action of the eyes, less tension in the jaws, more relaxation in the tongue and throat, and deeper breathing because of the effect of the new alignment on the diaphragm. There are also a sense of weightlessness and a diminution of the effort previously thought necessary to move one's limbs. Activity is now more free and flowing - no longer jerky and heavy with strain.*

Experimental Evidence

Professor Frank Pierce Jones, who was motivated to start a course of lessons due to fatigue and muscular aches, took up lessons with Alexander's brother Albert Redden Alexander, commonly known as A R. So impressed was he with the effects of the Technique that he not only took leave of absence from his post at Brown University in the US for three years while he trained as an Alexander teacher, but he researched the Technique scientifically at the Institute for Applied Experimental Psychology at Tufts University to discover what physical changes took place during Alexander lessons. During his research he used many techniques and instrumentation which included comparative psycho-physical reports, electromyography, multi-image photography, X-ray photography and a strain-gauge force-platform (a device to measure the force applied to a particular movement); an account of his experiments and their subsequent results may be found in his book *Body Awareness in Action*. Here he describes his first experience of the Technique:

> *I had expected something quite different - to have my faults of breathing and voice production diagnosed and to be given a set of exercises to correct them. Instead, Alexander chose the movement from sitting to standing for his demonstration. He made a few slight changes in the way I was sitting (they seemed quite arbitrary to me and I could not remember afterwards what they were), then, asking me to leave my head as it was, he initiated the upward movement without further instruction. Before I had a chance to organize my habitual response, the movement was completed and I found myself standing in a position that felt strangely comfortable. I was fully conscious throughout the movement and it was a consciousness, not of being moved by someone else ... but by a set of reflexes whose operation I knew nothing about.*
>
> *In addition to the reflex effect, the movement was notable for the way time and space were perceived. Though it took less time than usual to complete the movement, the rate at which I moved seemed paradoxically slower and more controlled and the trajectories that my head and trunk followed were unfamiliar. The impression was that of a sudden expansion in both dimensions, so that more time and space were available for the movement.*
>
> *The most striking aspect of the movement, however, was the sensory effect of lightness that it induced. The feeling had not been present at the start, nor had it been suggested to me; it was clearly*

a direct effect of the movement. After a short time the effect faded away, leaving me, however, with the certainty that I had glimpsed a new world of experience which had more to offer than the limited set of movement patterns, attitudes and responses to which I was accustomed.

Professor John Dewey, one of the founding fathers of scientific philosophy and modern education, was one of Alexander's first American pupils. The Technique influenced much of his writing:

Never before, I think, has there been such an acute consciousness of the failure of all external remedies as exist today, of the failure of all remedies and forces external to the individual man. It is, however, one thing to teach the need of a return to the individual man as the ultimate urgency in whatever mankind and society collectively can accomplish, to point out the necessity of straightening out this ultimate condition of whatever humanity in mass can obtain. It is another to discover the concrete procedure by which this greatest of all tasks can be executed. And this indispensable thing is exactly what Mr Alexander has accomplished. The discovery could not have been made and the method of procedure perfected except by dealing with adults who were badly co-ordinated. But the method is not one of remedy; it is one of constructive education. Its proper field of application is with the young, with the growing generation, in order that they may come to possess as early as possible in life a correct standard of sensory appreciation and self-judgement. When once a reasonably adequate part of a new generation has become properly co-ordinated, we shall have assurance for the first time that men and women in the future will be able to stand on their own feet, equipped with satisfactory psycho-physical equilibrium, to meet with readiness, confidence, and happiness instead of with

fear, confusion, and discontent, the bufferings and contingencies of
their surroundings.

Nobel Prize Winners

Over the years, people with substantial medical knowledge have also
spoken of the great benefits that the Alexander Technique can impart.
Sir Charles Sherrington, winner of the Nobel Prize for Medicine and
Physiology in the early part of this century, wrote:

> *Mr Alexander has done a service to the study of man by insistently*
> *treating each act as involving the whole integrated individual, the*
> *whole psycho-physical man. To take a step is an affair, not of this*
> *or that limb solely, but of the total neuro-muscular activity of the*
> *movement - not least of the head and neck.*

Professor Nikolaas Tinbergen, Nobel Prize-winner for Medicine
and Physiology in 1973, was so impressed with the Alexander
Technique that he dedicated a large proportion of his acceptance
speech to it. The following is an extract from that speech:

> *This story of perceptiveness, of intelligence, and of persistence*
> *shown by a man without medical training, is one of the true epics*
> *of medical research and practice. [He went on to say that through*
> *his own experience he had noted:] ... very striking improvements*
> *in such diverse things as high blood pressure, breathing, depth of*
> *sleep, overall cheerfulness, resilience against outside pressures, and*
> *in such a refined skill as playing a stringed instrument. So from*
> *personal experience we can already confirm some of the amazingly*
> *fantastic claims made by Alexander and his followers, namely, that*
> *many types of under-performance and even ailments, both mental*

and physical, can be alleviated, sometimes to a surprising extent,
by teaching the body musculature to function differently.

Support from the Medical Profession

Professor George Coghill, an anatomist and physiologist who spent 40 years studying the development and behaviour of animals and was considered one of the most outstanding scientists of this century, was another strong supporter of the Alexander Technique:

*It is my opinion that habitual use of improper reflex mechanisms
in sitting, standing and walking introduces conflict in the nervous
system, and that this conflict is the cause of fatigue and nervous
strain which bring ills in their train. Mr Alexander, by relieving this
conflict between the total pattern which is hereditary and innate,
and the reflex mechanisms which are individually cultivated, con-
serves the energies of the nervous system and by so doing corrects
not only postural difficulties, but also many other pathological
conditions that are not ordinarily recognized as postural. This is
a corrective principle that the individual learns for himself and is
the work of the self as a whole. It is not a system of physical culture
which involves only one system of organs for better or worse of the
economy of the whole organism. Mr Alexander's method lays hold
of the individual as a whole, as a self-vitalizing agent. He recondi-
tions and re-educates the reflex mechanisms and brings their habits
into normal relation with the functions of organisms as a whole. I
regard his method as thoroughly scientific and educationally sound.*

Raymond Dart, professor of anatomy at the University of Witwatersrand in South Africa and the world-famous anthropologist who discovered the first 'missing link' between man and his ape-like ancestors, also became fascinated with the Alexander Technique:

The electronic facilities [of electromyography and electroencepha-lography] have confirmed Alexander's insights and authenticated the technique he discovered in the 1890s of teaching both average and skilled adult individuals to become aware of their wrong body use, how to eliminate handicaps and thus achieve better (i.e. increasingly skilled) use of themselves, both physically and mentally.

Another of Alexander's medical admirers was Dr Wilfred Barlow, an Alexander teacher as well as a consultant rheumatologist:

In common with most doctors, my life has brought me into contact with many very intelligent people - many of them people of the highest talent. For what it is worth I must place on record that I found in Alexander an imaginative genius and an adherence to scientific method which I have not seen out-matched by anyone. I think he transformed the human condition although as yet on a tiny scale.

Even as far back as the 1920s a number of physicians and surgeons were urging the medical profession to take note of the valuable discoveries that had been made by Alexander. Nineteen of these professionals joined forces to write a letter to the British Medical Journal:

... As the medical men concerned we have observed the beneficial changes in use and functioning which have been brought about by the employment of Alexander's technique in the patients we have sent to him for help - even in the case of so called 'chronic disease'

- whilst those of us that have been his pupils have personally experienced equally beneficial results. We are convinced that 'an unsatisfactory manner of use, by interfering with general functioning, constitutes a predisposing cause of disorder and disease,' and that diagnosis of a patient's troubles must remain incomplete unless the medical man when making his diagnosis takes into consideration the influence of use upon functioning. Unfortunately, those responsible for the selection of subjects to be studied by medical students have not yet investigated the new field of knowledge and experience which has been opened up through Alexander's work, otherwise we believe that ere now the training necessary for acquiring this knowledge would have been included in the medical curriculum. To this end we beg to urge that as soon as possible steps should be taken for an investigation of Alexander's work and Technique ...

One of the doctors behind this letter was Peter Macdonald, who later became Chairman of the British Medical Association. This is an extract from his Inaugural Address:

Alexander is a teacher pure and simple. He does not profess to treat disease at all. If the manifestations of disease disappear in the process of education, well and good; if not the education of itself will have been worth while. Manifestations of disease, however, do disappear. Including myself, I know many of his pupils, some of them, like myself, medical men. I have investigated some of these cases, and I am talking about what I know ... there seemed to be a distinct betterment in cases of angina, pectoris, of asthma, of epilepsy, of tremor, of spinal curvature, and of difficulty of walking from locomotor ataxy, and from infantile paralysis. In short, I have seen, during the application of an educative process not directed to cure of disease, the manifestations of disease disappear, so that

I personally am convinced that Alexander is at least largely right when he says that disease is the result of wrong functioning. And further, I am beginning to wonder whether there are any manifestations of any forms of disease which may not disappear under a process of re-education on these lines ...

Randomised Controlled Trial

More recently, a major randomised, controlled clinical trial, funded by the Medical Research Council and the NHS, was carried out in the UK over a period of about six years. The aim of the trial (known as the ATEAM research) was to examine the effects of Alexander Technique lessons, exercise, and massage for chronic and recurrent back pain. The results of the trial, which were published in the British Medical Journal on 19th August 2008 (article reference BMJ 2008; 337:a884), clearly showed that Alexander Technique lessons give long-term benefit to chronic low-back pain sufferers. This multicentre trial involving 579 patients, led by GP researcher Professor Paul Little, University of Southampton, and GP Professor Debbie Sharp, Bristol University, is one of the few major studies to show significant long-term benefits for patients with chronic low-back pain. The trial assessed the benefits provided by Alexander Technique lessons, classical massage and normal GP care. Half the patients allocated to each intervention also received a GP prescription for general aerobic exercise.

The conclusions of the trial were that one-to-one lessons in the Alexander Technique from registered teachers have long-term benefits for patients with chronic back pain as the patients were reporting improvement long after the Alexander lessons, but not so with exercise or massage. These findings have led to improved understanding and acceptance of the Technique by the medical profession in recent years, and an increase in the number of doctors referring patients for Alexander Technique lessons.

A GP made the following comment:

From a discal neck injury in 1990 I developed progressive spinal problems. By 2002 I had suffered mechanical neck and back pain, several episodes of nerve root pain at different levels with loss of power and reflexes in my arms. I saw 4 neurosurgeons who all recommended different neck operations. I then developed complex regional pain syndrome and could barely use my right arm. I was in unbearable pain and virtually unable to move my neck. I started taking Alexander Technique lessons and began to experience improvement and lessening of pain after some 12-15 lessons. I did regular Alexander Technique for about 4 years. I have had progressive improvement since 2003 such that I now have no neck or arm pain. Alexander Technique lessons from a good teacher are an effective technique and were instrumental in my recovery. Based on simple applied principles it can afford sustained relief from pain of spinal origin. It teaches the body to undo neuromuscular tensions and reduce strain in normal motor function; probably cost effective were it taught in primary health care. I welcome this positive trial evidence.

Dr. Nick Mann GP

Full trial details can be seen on the British Medical Journal website: www.bmj.com/content/337/bmj.a884.full.

Our Supreme Inheritance

During his life, Alexander was not popular with everyone, as he had a reputation for challenging the status quo. He was a free thinker and his own individual character came out in his teaching; he also encouraged others to think for themselves rather than indiscriminately believing what other people told them instead of experiencing it for themselves. He depicted his Technique not as a physical method for curing ailments, but as a way of opening people's eyes and encouraging them to examine their individual human life in detail. Alexander was convinced that he had inadvertently stumbled upon the next stepping stone in man's evolutionary development: the power to reason clearly and thereby choose from a place of consciousness. He claimed to offer the key that released human beings from the chains of ignorance and suffering into a more vigilant existence - a way that offered a deliberate control over the instincts, emotions and unrestrained mind which had been the cause of man's irrational behaviour throughout the ages. He maintained that as a result of practising his Technique, stress, disharmony and unhappiness would naturally be eradicated, allowing people to feel free from erroneous concepts and faulty perceptions about what is important in life, and from the 'mind-wandering' which so often controls everything that people do and say.

Hint

As our entrenched habits gradually become weaker they are replaced with greater conscious control, which allows us to let go of prejudices and conditioned ideas about what we should be achieving in our lives, and instead experiencing life for what it is.

Alexander Lessons

It is important to realize that when we embark on this journey to self-fulfilment we will be dealing with habitual behaviour patterns that may have developed over many years and which have hindered our emotional development, preventing free expression of our true personality. These habits serve as a protection in situations where we feel vulnerable or insecure. The aim of Alexander Technique lessons is not to try to strip us of this emotional 'armouring' as long as it is fulfilling its purpose, but to bring about a process of change which replaces our old, inflexible, outworn habits with a new way of being which is more appropriate and adaptable to the ever-changing world in which we live. This process of change does not take place unconsciously, but is directed by our own superior intelligence, which guides us towards the best development of our own unique personality. It is important to realize that although some of the sensations experienced during this process may be unexpected or feel unfamiliar, this is a necessary accompaniment to positive change.

When we stop being swept along by the circumstances that we have been conditioned to believe are important, we begin to get a true perspective on life and may very well wonder why we have not taken the necessary steps to reduce stress before. It comes as a great relief to realize that happiness is not a matter of externals, but a feeling within us that we carry wherever we go.

Priorities

Helen Keller, the deaf and blind poet, once said that the best and most beautiful things in the world cannot be seen, nor touched, but are felt in the heart. If we are ever to feel our true beauty, it is essential that each of us realizes who we really are, rather than believing what everyone else has taught us to be. In our heart of hearts we all know that there is something very wrong with the values and priorities that society has imposed on us.

If you suffer from stress, panic attacks, anxiety or depression this is a clear sign that your priorities in life are out of balance and that changes are urgently needed. If the habit of stress has been strongly reinforced over many years, which is often the case due to the 'end-gaining' way in which most of us live, you will be out of touch with what you really need and what your heart is trying to communicate to you. But no amount of Alexander lessons or inspirational quotations will help you to reduce stress - you must decide for yourself to re-evaluate the priorities in your life.

It is so often the case that we freely give our valuable time to the trivial things in life while at the same time placing hardly any significance on the things that truly matter. The realization that our time on this planet is limited, and that we cannot take anything with us when we die, can encourage us to look seriously at these priorities and help us to live life in the present rather than to be so goal-orientated. Just before his death, the famous warrior Alexander the Great saw the foolishness of his actions and ordered the following epitaph for his grave:

> Here lies Alexander the Great,
> who set out to conquer the whole world,
> came into this world empty handed
> also left empty handed.

Legend has it that he instructed some of his loyal subjects to make sure that his empty hands were extended out from either side of the coffin to demonstrate this fact. This great conqueror left this message in the hope that those who came after him would realize the folly of living life for material gain.

Once we start to appreciate our own individual qualities we no longer need to compare ourselves with other people, and we begin to measure our success by what we are rather than by our worldly achievements. As a result, the stress and irritation that we often feel begins to be replaced by a deep contentment, inner harmony and love of life.

Tip

Since our actions can only take place in the here and now, being aware of the way we move encourages us to be in the present rather than think about 'what could be' and 'what if'.

Entelechy - Your Hidden Potential

The Alexander Technique gives you the power to alter your consciousness and allow a spontaneous gratitude to take place; since the source of this consciousness has no limits there is no end to how attentive or appreciative you can be. The more aware you are, the more alive you will feel and the greater your capacity to enjoy life. As the process of change starts to take place, stress, fear and worry are put in their proper place in the overall scheme of things.

By beginning to understand and put into practice the principles behind Alexander's teachings, you will be able to change the habitual reactions and responses which are the root cause of muscle tension, mental worries and emotional instability. By learning different responses, first by inhibiting and secondly by conscious choice, you can start to dissolve mental turmoil and feel the peace that, although often obscured, has always been present within you. As your stress levels are reduced you will be able to reconnect with your true self and get a better sense of what you really want out of life.

The word *entelechy* comes from the Greek and means 'the actualization or manifestation of a hidden potential'. In each and every one of us lies the possibility to become something more than we think we are - in fact we have far greater potential than we can ever imagine. However, it takes great courage to welcome the metamorphosis that makes this potential our reality.

Hint

The biggest step to eliminating stress from your life is to give up trying to get it right.

Tip

Appreciation and enjoyment of life are the natural antidotes to the stresses and strains of modern living.

Obtaining lasting happiness does not involve grasping for peace and contentment, but weeding out those things in life that prevent inner happiness from emerging. There is *absolutely nothing you need to do*; but there are plenty of behaviour patterns, faulty ways of thinking and erroneous judgements about ourselves and others that we need to nip in the bud. When, through awareness and conscious choice we have the ability to refuse to become stressed when demands are placed upon us, we will begin to become aware of how incredible we are and how beautiful life really can be. This is our supreme inheritance and it can be realized by any human being - the only requirements are to be courageous enough to be proved wrong, to be daring enough to let go of lifelong habits and to have enough determination to refuse to be swept along by the madness of this world. The reward that awaits us is a feeling of love - the love that is right behind each breath that you take.

In one of his most powerful writings, Alexander points directly and clearly to what we need to do in order to claim this supreme inheritance:

> *It is essential that the people of civilization should comprehend the value of their inheritance, that outcome of the long process of evolution which will enable them to govern the uses of their own physical mechanisms. By and through consciousness and the application of a reasoning intelligence, man may rise above the powers of all disease and physical disabilities. This triumph is not to be won in sleep, in trance, in submission, in paralysis, or in anaesthesia, but in a clear, open-eyed, reasoning, deliberate consciousness and apprehension of the wonderful potentialities possessed by mankind, the transcendent inheritance of a conscious mind.*

The Miracle Within

I would like to leave you with this true story. It tells of a lame beggar in India who, because of his disability, slept, ate and begged in exactly the same place each day. For many years he received barely getting enough rupees to feed himself. Then one day he died, and because he had no family in the village the local people had to decide what to do with him. After some discussion they decided to bury him on the very spot where he had spent the last three decades begging, so they started to dig a grave. After a short while they found a large box two feet under the surface; when they opened it they found it was full of gold, silver and priceless jewels. As it turned out the beggar had spent all his life begging for a few rupees when he was, in fact, sitting on a priceless treasure. In the same way, each of us contains, within ourselves, a priceless treasure, if we can only recognize it for what it is. The Alexander Technique is a tool which can help you to discover your birthright: to have true joy in your heart. These words of Donald Walters describe well the experience of joy:

> True joy is not an emotional state.
> It is not that which one feels when some desire is satisfied,
> or when everything at last goes well ...
> It is inward; it is of the soul.

This life is full of wonderful opportunities, magic and miracles - all we need to do is let go of our fear and allow life to unfold without interference. This is the highest of all human achievements.

Useful Addresses

Richard Brennan's websites with useful articles and information about the Alexander Technique:

www.alexander.ie

www.alexandertechniqueireland.com

Details of good quality **wedge cushions** for cars and chairs (but not for sofas).

www.alexander.ie/cushion.html

Details of **footwear** designed with the Alexander Technique in mind:

www.vivobarefoot.com

www.terraplana.com/vivobarefoot_benefits.php

Direction Magazine is a wonderful resource for articles and information, for both teachers and students of the Alexander Technique. Visit the website for free audios, articles, live interviews plus 25 years of back issues in stock.

www.directionjournal.com

Alexander Technique Societies Worldwide

The International Societies of Teachers of the Alexander Technique below give details of how to find a teacher near you. All teachers listed on these websites have undergone extensive three year training.

UK

Website for teachers who are members of the Society of Teachers of the Alexander Technique (STAT), the first and longest-established Alexander Technique organisation. Teachers listed are mainly from the UK and Ireland, but also include many other countries. (For Ireland please also see ISATT below).

www.stat.org.uk

AUSTRALIA

Australian Society of Teachers of the Alexander Technique (AuSTAT).

www.austat.org.au

BELGIUM

Belgian Association of teachers of the Alexander Technique (AEFMAT).

www.fmalexandertech.be

BRAZIL

Associacao Brasileira de Tecnica Alexander (ABTA).

www.abtalexander.com.br

CANADA

Canadian Society of Teachers of the F. M. Alexander Technique/ Société Canadienne des Professeurs de la Technique F. M. Alexander (CANSTAT).

www.canstat.ca

DENMARK

Dansk forening af lærere i Alexanderteknik (DFLAT).
www.dflat.dk

FINLAND

Suomen Alexander-tekniikan Opettajat (FINSTAT).
www.finstat.fi

FRANCE

L'Association Francaise des Professeurs de La Technique Alexander
-(APTA).
www.techniquealexander.info

GERMANY

Alexander Technik Verband Deutschland (ATVD)
www.alexander-technik.org

IRELAND

The Irish Society of Alexander Technique Teachers (ISATT).
www.isatt.ie

ISRAEL

The Israeli Society of Teachers of the Alexander Technique.
www.alexander.org.il

NETHERLANDS

Nederlandse Vereniging van Leraren in de Alexander Techniek (NeVLAT).
www.alexandertechniek.nl

NEW ZEALAND

Alexander Technique Teachers' Society of New Zealand (ATTSNZ).
www.alexandertechnique.org.nz

NORWAY

Norsk Forening for Laerere i Alexanderteknikk (NFLAT).
www.alexanderteknikk.no

SOUTH AFRICA

South African Society of Teachers of the Alexander Technique (SASTAT).
www.alexandertechnique.org.za

SPAIN

Spanish Society of Teachers of the Alexander Technique (APTAE).
www.aptae.net

SWITZERLAND

Schweizerischer Verband der Lehrerinnen und Lehrer der F.M. Alexander-Technik (SVLAT/ASPITA).
www.alexandertechnik.ch

USA

American Society for the Alexander Technique AmSAT.
www.alexandertech.org

Other interesting websites

www.alexandertechnique.org/info.html
www.alexandertechnique.com
www.ati-net.com
www.atcongress.com

Further Reading

Easy-to-follow and informative books on the Alexander Technique:

• Brennan, Richard, *The Alexander Technique - New Perspectives*, *Chrysalis Books 2001*

• —, *The Alexander Technique Manual, Little Brown 1996*

• —, *The Alexander Technique Workbook, Collins and Brown 2011*

• —, *Improve Your Posture with the Alexander Technique, Duncan Baird Publishers 2011*

• *Chance, Jeremy, The Alexander Technique, Thorsons 1998*

• *Gelb, Michael, Body Learning, Aurum Press 1981*

• *Stevens, Chris, The Alexander Technique, Optima 1987*

• *Carolyn Nicholls, Body, Breath and Being, D &B Publishing 2008*

• *Park, Glen, The Art of Changing, Ashgrove Press 1989*

More in-depth or specialized books on the Alexander Technique:

• *Macdonald, Patrick, The Alexander Technique as I See It, Sussex Academic Press: 1989*

• *Marjorie Barlow, An Examined Life, Mornum Time Press 2002*

• *Carrington, Walter, Thinking Aloud, Mornum Time Press 1994*

• *Heirich Jane, Voice and the Alexander Technique, Mornum Time Press 2004*

- *Westfeldt, Lulie, Alexander, F. Matthias, The Man and his Work, Centerline Press 1964*

- *Barlow, Wilfred, The Alexander Principle, Gollancz 1973*

- *Conable, Barbara and William, How to learn the Alexander Technique, Andover Press 1991*

- *Maisel, Edward, The Resurrection of the Body, Shambala 1969*

- *Pierce Jones, Frank, Body Awareness in Action / The Freedom to Change, Shocken Books 1976*

- *Missy Vineyard, How you Stand, How you Move, How you Live, Morlowe and Company 2007*

Books by F.M. Alexander himself (some of which are difficult to follow due to his style of writing):

- *Alexander, F.M., The Use of the Self, Gollancz 1985*

- *—, The Universal Constant in Living, Centerline Press 1986*

- *—, Man's Supreme Inheritance, Centerline Press 1988*

- *—, Conscious Control of the Individual, Gollancz 1987*

The Alexander Self Help CD& MP3

The CD (or MP3) is the perfect accompaniment to this book. It is designed to be used when doing the lying down exercise (chapter 3) and gives clear and concise instructions on:

• How to eliminate unwanted tension.

• How to prevent or relieve back pain.

• How to improve your breathing.

• How to reduce your stress levels.

• How to clear your mind from unwanted thoughts.

• How to practice the two Alexander principles of Inhibition and Direction.

• How to stay in the present moment.

This CD costs £10.00, US$18 or €15, including postage & packing, and is available from:

Richard Brennan
The Alexander Technique Centre,
Kirkullen Lodge, Tooreeny, Moycullen,
Co Galway, Republic of Ireland.
Tel: +353 91 555800
Email: info@alexander.ie

It can also be downloaded (MP3 format) or purchased online at www.alexander.ie.
Other books, posture improving chairs and stools, and wedge-shaped cushions are also available from this website. A

Index

A
actors 148
adolescents 95, 134, 145
adrenal glands 56, 93
adrenaline 4, 56, 57, 103
advertisements 10, 25
affection 23
aggression 20
alcohol 20
Alexander, Albert Redden 156
Alexander, F. Matthias 23, 27, 33-49, 52, 136, 157-162, 166
Alexander Technique, history of the 33-49
Alexander Technique lessons 40, 68, 101-111, 124-126, 147, 156
Alexander the Great 163, 164
anger 4, 10, 127, 130-132, 154
angina 155
anti-depressants 3, 126
anxiety 2, 3, 7, 20, 89-111, 115, 148
appetite, loss of 115
appreciation 21, 23, 73, 129, 136, 137, 164, 165
Aristotle 127
arteries, hardening of 59
arthritis 53
asthma 8, 33, 44, 53, 54, 58, 147, 148, 161
arguments 130-134
Augustine, Saint 140
Austin, Dr John 104
awareness 27, 28, 63, 103, 104, 121, 140, 148-151, 164, 165

B
backache 8, 44, 52, 53, 58, 62, 73
Bach, Richard 101
Barlow, Dr Wilfred 104, 147, 148, 159, 160
balance 40, 43, 94, 126, 137
behaviour patterns 20, 23, 61, 116, 117, 157-162, 165
blame 115, 134

blood circulation 53, 54
blood clotting 53, 60
blood sugar 56, 57, 93
breathing 23, 43, 57, 60, 93, 104, 123, 130, 139-152, 155, 158
breathing exercises 147, 148
breathing problems 8, 55, 92
British Medical Journal 160
British Medical Association 160
Bronowski, Dr. Jacob 46

C
cancer 53, 76, 77
Carnegie, Dale 73
Carrel, Dr Alexis 73
car-seats 17
cause and effect 37, 90
chairs 15-17
chemical causes of depression 118
children 11-21, 134
Christmas 24, 25
choice 27
cholesterol 57, 59
Churchill, Sir Winston 48
circumstances 126, 163
city life 4
Coghill, Professor George 158
colds 52, 53
common sense 27
computers 5
confidence 15, 21, 22, 54, 91, 157
constipation 54
conscious control 7, 27, 47, 50, 132, 155, 162, 165, 166
co-ordination 40, 82, 92, 95, 126, 157
coronary thrombosis 54
cortisol 56
criticism 21
Cummins Anna 137

D
Dart, Professor Raymond 159
deadlines 6, 10
depression 2, 7, 8, 20, 113-126
Dewey, Professor John 32, 157
diabetes 8, 53, 59
digestive disorders 8, 53-55
Directions 42-45, 65, 66, 85, 86, 102-105, 122, 123, 137
disempowerment 25

divorce 4, 10, 117
dizziness 55, 92

E
education, general 12, 155
education, personal 31, 32, 155-161
epilepsy 161
Emerson, Ralph Waldo 23, 69
emotional armouring 162
emotions 20, 32, 114, 117, 127-137, 161
end-gaining 8, 24, 150
endocrine glands 56
endorphins 59
enjoyment of life 22
environment reaction to our 4, 10-12, 24, 28-30, 49, 73, 80
exhaustion 56-58, 129
experimental evidence 104, 156

F
fatigue 8, 55-57, 130, 159
failure, fear of 97, 98
faulty sensory perception 38, 39, 49, 62, 136, 137, 151
fear 5, 11, 15, 21, 46, 55, 60, 82, 91-101, 157
fear reflex 7, 55-60
feelings, talking about 120, 130-134
fibromyalgia 8
fight or flight response 7, 55-60, 82, 93, 102
flu 52
freedom of choice 13, 25-27, 50, 86, 152
Freud Sigmund 46
fulfilment 75, 81, 162
future, fear of the 79

G
Garlick, Dr David 104
goal-orientated 8, 23, 45, 49
Goleman, Daniel 20, 131
gratitude 136, 137, 164, 165
gravity 43, 64, 150
guilt 21, 114

H
habits 7, 9, 35, 36, 45-48, 82, 83, 93, 105, 145, 162
happiness 2, 22, 24, 27, 28, 72, 81, 137, 157, 163
harmony 28, 30
headaches 8, 52-55, 58, 73
heartburn 54

heart problems 2, 6, 8, 55, 59, 60, 74, 131, 155
heart rate, increase of 56, 57, 59, 92, 93, 130, 131
Hopi Indians 132-133
hormones 7, 8, 55-57, 93, 131
horses 33
Huxley, Aldous 32, 154, 155
hypertension (high blood pressure) 8, 54, 57, 59, 73, 158
hyperventilation 54, 60
hypothalamus 56

I
immune system 53, 56
indigestion 54, 59
insomnia 11, 58, 70, 115
infectious diseases 52-55, 58
inhibition 46-50, 82, 83, 132-137, 155, 165
insulin 59
intelligence 23
irritation 4, 57, 130
isolation 95, 114

K
Keller, Helen 113, 163
kinaesthetic sense 62
kindness 74
Krishnamurti 8

J
Jones, Professor Frank Pierce 46, 156, 157
joy 152, 167

L
Lao Tse 153
larynx 36-41, 48
laughter 23, 119
lethargy 57, 115
Lewinsohn, Peter 114
life, the pace of 30
life-force 139, 140
lifestyle 11, 30
lightness 106
longevity 73
loneliness 114
love 74, 99, 129, 166
lungs 141, 150

M
MacArthur, General 121
Maisel, Edward 155
marriage 4, 22, 137
materialism 5, 8, 164
McEwen, Bruce 53
meditation 154
metabolism 56, 58
migraines 8, 52, 53, 58, 73
Milton, John 76
mind, the power of the 76-79, 88
mind wandering 86, 121, 162
misuse of the body 36, 49, 141
movement, ease of 12, 26, 27, 37-43, 106, 155
muscular tension 3, 7, 15, 52, 57, 63, 73, 82, 102, 105, 130, 136, 141,
muscular system 31, 82, 93, 101, 141
musicians 148

N
neck problems 8, 53
negative thinking 11, 121
nervous disorders 73, 89-111
nervous system 54, 58, 101, 102, 159
neuro-muscular system 10, 93
Nobel prize 73, 158
noise 4, 10
noradrenalin 56

O
obligations 26
openness 13
over-active mind 63, 64

P
panic attacks 8, 90-111
Partridge, Sibyl 86
peace 30, 165
pelvis 17, 41, 44, 64
personality traits 11
physical causes of depression 116
physiological causes of depression 117
physiological changes during stress 55-60, 91-93
pituitary gland 56
Plato 32, 119
play 23
pollution 4
posture 5, 13-17, 27, 44, 45, 54, 61-63, 114-119, 141-145

prejudices 31, 49
pregnancy 10
present, living in the 71-81, 85-88
pressure 21, 22, 128
priorities 74, 75, 163, 164
Primary Control, The 37-39, 93-95, 102, 122
Primary Directions 42-44, 102
psychotherapy 119, 154
psycho-physical equilibrium 157
pushchairs 17

Q
quality of life 1-28, 77, 135

R
Ram Dass 89
reason 27, 46, 166
re-education 49, 101, 159
reflexes 62, 122, 152, 156, 159
relationships 4, 22, 128-133, 137
repetitive strain injury 53
respiratory system 141, 145, 146, 152
respiratory problems 33, 147
responses 9, 11, 41-48
responsibility 26, 98, 99, 125, 134
relaxation 22, 146, 152
ribs 104, 141, 149
ridicule 21
risks, taking 119, 120

S
school 12-19, 60, 61, 95, 97, 117
Secondary Directions 44, 45
self-discovery 24, 30
self-esteem 21, 22, 99, 117, 128, 129
Selye, Hans 56
semi-supine position 64-68
sex drive, loss of 55
sex hormones 56
shame 21, 95
Shaw, George Bernard 32, 126, 155
Sherrington, Sir Charles 158
skin problems 8
sleep 11, 55, 67, 70, 110, 115
Smiles, Samuel 29
spine 17, 43, 145, 161
spontaneity 71, 164

standing, release of tension while 45
Stair Nadine 74
Stevens, Chris 104
stimuli 22, 41, 48
stress, effects of 51-68
stress management 7
stress, reduction of 26, 58-61, 64, 163
strokes 2, 59, 60, 74
success 23, 46, 167
Sullivan, Michael 15

T
Tagore, Rahbindranath 139
Talmud 136
technology 3
television 5, 10, 63
tension 23, 31, 42, 148
tension, release of 42-45, 85, 109, 110, 126, 148, 154
testosterone 56
Thoreau, Henry David 1
thought patterns 42
thyroxine 56, 58
Tinbergen, Professor Nikolaas 158
tiredness 8, 55-57
traffic 4, 10
tranquillisers 6, 99

U
ulcers 8, 54, 59, 74
unemployment 83, 117, 129
unity of body, mind and emotions 32, 45, 49, 77-79, 96, 146, 147

V
violence 10, 130
voice problems 24, 33-37, 47

W
Walters, Donald 167
whispered 'ah' procedure 150-151
Wilde Stuart 128
words 132-133
World Health Organization 114
worry 2, 7, 20, 69-88